LINDA MASON'S
SUN-SIGN
MAKEOVERS

LINDA MASON'S SUN-SIGN MAKEOVERS

PREFACE BY SHIRLEY LORD

Farrar, Straus and Giroux
New York

a very special thanks to

George, Daniel, Melodie, Sylko, Yvonne, Sophie, Shirley, Jody, Marshall, Roger Durrieu of Universal Model Agency, and Pamela of Paris Planning for their unfailing encouragement

Copyright © 1985 by Linda Mason
Preface copyright © 1985 by Shirley Lord
All rights reserved
Library of Congress catalog card number: 85-80126
Published simultaneously in Canada by
Collins Publishers, Toronto
Printed in the United States of America
by General Offset Company, Inc.

Designed by Patricia Manzone
First edition, 1985

To Mam and Dad

Preface

I frequently borrow—for speeches, both public and private—one of Sir Winston Churchill's favorite sayings. "Ma'am, I do believe we're all worms," he told his startled dinner companion back in the thirties. "But I also believe I'm a glowworm!" As a journalist who graduated at an early age from London's Street of Ink, Fleet Street, I'm a firm believer in worms and glowworms. I've seen for myself how natural talent *shines* out of people... as it shines out of the author of this book, the world-renowned makeup artist Linda Mason.

I first met Linda when, for five years, I left the world of newspapers and magazines to become vice president of Helena Rubinstein, where I created programs and promotions to sell Rubinstein products worldwide. I chose experts in all fields of beauty and fitness to assist me, but none was as enthusiastic and as innovative as Linda Mason. In two programs that I devised, the Beauty Breakfast and the Better Look Program, the grand finale—when Linda performed a transformation act with Rubinstein cosmetics—was "the best part," most women would say. It was as good as having Houdini up on stage, with one major difference: unlike the magician, Linda explained how she achieved her color magic step by step.

The largest promotion of my Helena Rubinstein career involved Silk Fashion, a line of beauty products which actually contained silk fibers. I "built" a spectacular "laboratory" in one of the magnificent reception rooms at the Villa d'Este on Lake Como (home of the silk kings of Italy), where the press, goggle-eyed, watched the product come into being, from live silkworms spinning silk at one end of the room to the final package at the other. But again, where were the traffic jams? In the next reception room, where Linda showed how even great beauties like Elsa Martinelli and Veruschka could be made to glow with the Silk Fashion colors.

In my present capacity as Director of Beauty and Fitness for *Vogue*, I can say without hesitation that Linda Mason is one of our most trusted and inspired makeup artists. Working with *Vogue*'s top models, she creates looks that often trigger cosmetics manufacturers to introduce new colors or color combinations. I also happen to share Linda's fascination with and belief in the study of astrology. From time to time, when our frantic schedules permit, Linda comes over to my apartment to "transform" me for an important event. I always mean to watch her closely, but somehow I never do. Perhaps it's because my Virgo sensibility takes for granted that my face is in the best hands I can find... perhaps it's because my moon in (caring/emotional) Cancer means I have to catch up with what is happening in Linda's life, while my (happy-go-lucky) Sagittarius ascendant means I like to open a bottle of good wine when Linda is there and turn the makeover hour into a party... perhaps it's also because Linda's hands relax me so beautifully. Now, with this book's help, I hope to be able to achieve the same extraordinary results by myself.

I am proud to count myself as an early supporter of this book—in my opinion, a solid work on a neglected aspect of beauty. Unusual? Yes, but as you turn the pages, full of common-sense ideas illustrated in the most substantial way, you will see how our sun signs do indeed influence our features, which, with the right makeup, can be developed into *star* qualities!

Shirley Lord

Introduction

My interest in makeup began when I was a child, watching my feminine Pisces mother taking so much care with her appearance. She made it seem such a wonderfully magical thing, as all Pisces have the knack of doing. My interest reached its peak when I first worked in Paris, a city ruled by my sun sign, Virgo. The well-known perfectionism of Virgo nearly guarantees success in a career which demands so much attention to detail. From the subtly made up, perfectionist Parisian women, I received not only professional inspiration but also the first indication that national characteristics are influenced by the zodiac.

The intuitive qualities of Cancer, my rising sign, have made me more understanding of the needs of the beauty editors, photographers, and designers with whom I've collaborated, and is responsible for the protective, motherly feelings I have for the models. The three planets I have in Libra—Mars, Jupiter, and Neptune—have inspired my love of color. And my moon in Aries has made me more outgoing and outspoken—characteristics necessary for sharing ideas with those around me.

In addition, there are interesting conclusions to be drawn about the various sun signs' approach to modeling. Two of the top runway models, Pat Cleveland and Jerry Hall, were born under the feminine, sexy sign of Cancer. It takes a long time and a lot of subtle flattery to gain the Cancerian's confidence, yet a certain firmness is necessary—otherwise, she would run rings around you. An Aries is very easy to identify, not only because of her lithe body but also because of her commanding, gregarious manner. If you can get her to sit still, she's wonderful to work with. Gemini and Pisces make excellent models, but for very different reasons: Pisces is malleable and has a sensitivity and sensuality that are highly photogenic; Gemini, epitomized by Brooke Shields, has great natural beauty and superb bone structure. Scorpios are strong and secure, and at times have a little difficulty accepting certain things asked of them. Part of the problem lies in their makeup. It needs to be only half as strong as that of other signs, but most makeup artists don't realize this. Libras are so artistic themselves that they have trouble accepting anything less than perfect, which can lead to difficulty in the modeling profession. Taurus (the other sign governed by Venus, the goddess of beauty) is found mainly in the fashion show, since photographic modeling is too abstract for this earth sign. There aren't many Virgo models; Virgos intellectualize and as a result have difficulty letting go in front of the camera. Until recently, there were few Capricorn models. Fashion leaned more toward the relaxed, smiling Sagittarius style, while Capricorn is more sensuous and serious. That has changed completely; now cool, captivating Capricorn is one of the most popular models.

The Leo woman is seldom found modeling. This is a fixed sign and Leo often has difficulty seeing herself other than she is. She also likes to command, and the role of the model does not allow for leadership. It is in the air sign Aquarius, however, that we find the best, most adaptable models—though not necessarily easy to make up, as their eyes are difficult. Aquarius is willing to try anything, for she has the ability to see herself objectively, and is unthreatened by transformation. She is totally interested and at ease.

Knowledge of astrology has enhanced my relationships with designers as well as with models. The easy, flowing Virgo/Taurus relationship was realized in Paris with Jean-Paul Gaultier. Our professional rapport was effortless in part because he likes makeup that is typically Taurean, with earthy, sensual colors, and I could easily understand the preferences of my fellow earth sign. More effort was necessary with Thierry Mugler (Sagittarius), but in the end it was most rewarding. Thierry has an excellent understanding of makeup and he taught me an enormous amount, especially as I watched his style evolve from a strong, sculptured look to a softer, more feminine quality. Anne Marie Beretta helped me perfect my Oriental-look makeup. This is her favorite style, which is unsurprising, since Libra, her sign, rules Japan. Her makeup is always elegant and well balanced, with unbroken lines lengthening the delicate eyes. This accentuates the mysterious total effect of the clothing and makeup.

It has been with the water signs that I have felt the most freedom in my work. With the late France Andrevie (Cancer), no words seemed necessary, perhaps because of my Cancer rising. We had an intuitive understanding of each other's needs, and an almost uncanny ability to stimulate each other professionally. As a result, she has allowed me to do some of my most creative work, never worrying about potentially strong reactions to my more daring ideas. With Scorpio Rei Kawakubo (of Comme des Garçons), I felt a similar liberating sensation which inspired me to explore and experiment. Here the makeup was minimalistic.

Two Pisces designers were extremely gratifying to work with, for different reasons. Willi Smith of WilliWear created an electric atmosphere with his fun, easy-to-wear clothes. I was virtually free of restrictions in my work with him and the makeup that emerged from our collaboration was modern and carefree. Perry Ellis, on the other hand, was a more typical Pisces, favoring a feminine, dreamlike style. (One of his favorite models, Lise Ryall, is also a Pisces.)

Ideas flowed easily with fellow Virgo Stephen Sprouse. He is extremely quick-minded, and his unusual clothes make strong statements. A perfectionist—once again, typical of the sign.

Working with so many people under such intense circumstances—at crowded fashion shows, at 4 a.m. by candlelight in the jungle, and under a palm tree in 110-degree heat—has taught me a great deal about personality differences, and the patterns that emerged have helped me develop my theory of astrological influences as they apply to makeup.

Linda Mason

Why Sun-Sign Makeup?

Early in my career as a makeup artist, I began to notice striking physical similarities in women of the same birth sign. There are certain physiognomic traits characteristic of each sign, but even when these traits are not outstanding, personality, taste, and styles of self-expression combine to produce strong likenesses. The characteristics that differentiate women of various sun signs obviously form part of each woman's special attraction, and it soon becomes clear that this innate appeal can be enhanced by makeup colors and techniques geared to each individual sign.

In *Linda Mason's Sun-Sign Makeovers*, I've presented the forms, colors, and techniques which I consider flattering to each particular sign. There are easy step-by-step instructions illustrated with before-and-after photographs of twenty-eight women. Each has a large variety of beauty problems well within the range of ordinary good looks. You'll find that makeup specifically designed for their signs has transformed them all into stunning—and highly individual—women.

Each chapter begins with a basic description of the physical characteristics that I find common to those born under that sign, and some general guidelines involving the most flattering colors and techniques for each. These are followed by makeovers which apply these guidelines and which, with detailed instructions, can serve as a perfect introduction to your sun sign's makeup. You might also draw an idea or two from another sign's makeover and improvise a bit, to create the effect that you feel best expresses *your* nature. Don't forget to consider your rising sign and planetary influences, as they can be extremely strong.

For additional help, there is a detailed technical index at the back of the book. It explains basic techniques, such as applying lipstick and plucking eyebrows, and will tell you in which chapter you'll find help for specific flaws. It will also direct you to particular color schemes you might like to try. Quite possibly there are several makeovers in other chapters which can be modified for your own sun sign. As long as the final result conforms to your nature rather than masks it, you should experiment freely. It's the best way to discover.

Makeup will always be an important form of communication. To communicate properly, it's essential to understand—and appreciate—your own personality and unique beauty, and learn to present them as effectively as possible. *Linda Mason's Sun-Sign Makeovers* is designed to help every woman, beautiful in her own way, look her absolute best.

L. M.

Contents

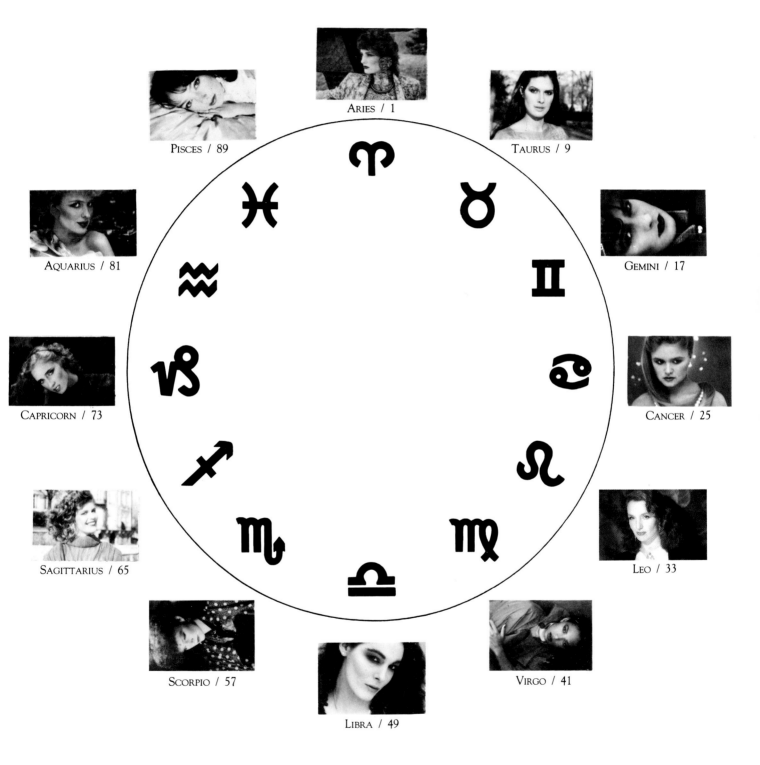

LINDA MASON'S
SUN-SIGN
MAKEOVERS

a r i e s
m a r c h 21 — a p r i l 20

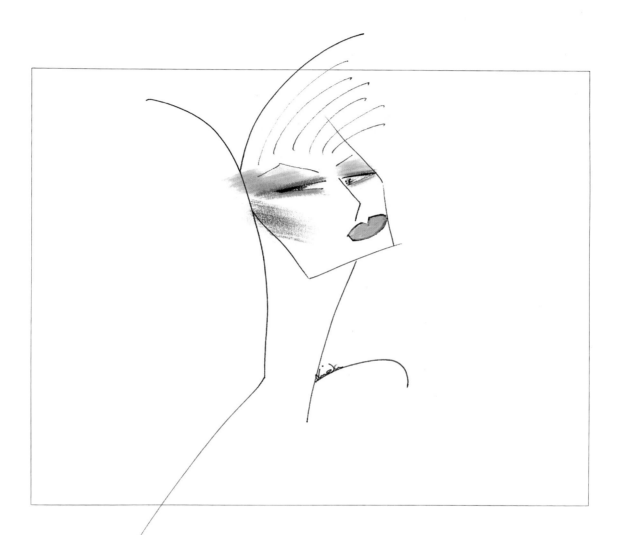

Aries' strikingly handsome face is one of the most easily recognized in the zodiac. The determined features are usually sharp, never soft or blurred, with eyes small enough to make the beautifully defined mouth seem quite large in comparison. The Aries forehead can be flat and low; high prominent cheekbones form the widest part of this flat-planed face. The eyebrows of the brunette Aries are most often heavy, while those of the blonde are fine and well shaped. In profile, the nose quite often has a slight bump just beneath the bridge.

When Mars, the ruling planet, is strong in Aries, there is a reddish glow to the hair and face; still, the complexion is usually strong, smooth, and of even coloring. She loves the sun and tans easily, which is fortunate, since the impatient Aries is not one to bother with suntan lotion.

Beneath her somewhat masculine exterior, Aries is all woman. She appreciates makeup but does not have time to play with it. Browsing through beauty shops is not a favorite pastime of this energetic sign—she can be seen rushing into a store with a nearly finished product, buying the same thing, and rushing out again. In a similar way, she rarely experiments with color and stays with the same makeup over a long period of time. Since Aries is such a forceful, modern personality, however, she can keep the same look forever and never appear dated.

Aries should stay away from bright, contrasty colors, unless that color is red, which is very flattering on her sensual lips. Red can even be used on the eyes, as an alternative to her usual neutral shades.

For her eyes, the best choice is black, even for blondes, with gray or brown a close second. There should be little or no shine in the shadow, and the color should be quite deep to help balance the size of the eyes with that of the mouth. Black or brown liner applied right next to the lashes will also enlarge the eyes, especially if they are dark.

A light, neutral beige foundation, more golden than pink, best enhances Aries' strong, healthy complexion. Over this, the most flattering blushers are those of neutral shades, such as beige, russet, or muted

pink. Light peaches and pinks should be avoided, as they are too soft and romantic for this tomboyish sign. The blusher should be applied directly on the prominent Aries cheekbones.

Apart from the red already mentioned, lipstick colors should remain neutral. All shades of beige, pale or muted dark pinks, and clear or colored lip gloss are complimentary to her makeup colors and her style. As a novelty, and to break the monotony of the other more conservative shades in her makeup, a metallic copper or metalized gray lipstick, or a brown shade—even quite dark—would be stunning and dramatic. The more feminine, frosted lipsticks, however, should never be used.

The bloodstone, the diamond, and all metals of a reddish hue, especially copper, are ruled by Aries. Worn separately or together, they are the most flattering jewelry for her strong beauty. Thick copper necklaces in particular look superb on her long slender neck, enhancing the bold sensuality of this fire sign.

lilo

To modify: The small eyes
To accentuate: The beautifully shaped sensuous mouth
The high cheekbones

1. Apply a *yellow-tinted beige foundation* (not pink) over the entire face, including eyelids.

2. With a *black kohl pencil*, lightly shade the base of the bottom lashes, the outer corner of the upper eye at the

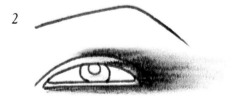

2

base of the lashes, and the eye socket. Blend outward.

3. Powder face and eyelids with *transparent powder.*

4. Apply *taupe powder eye shadow* to the eyelid, blending it into the kohl.

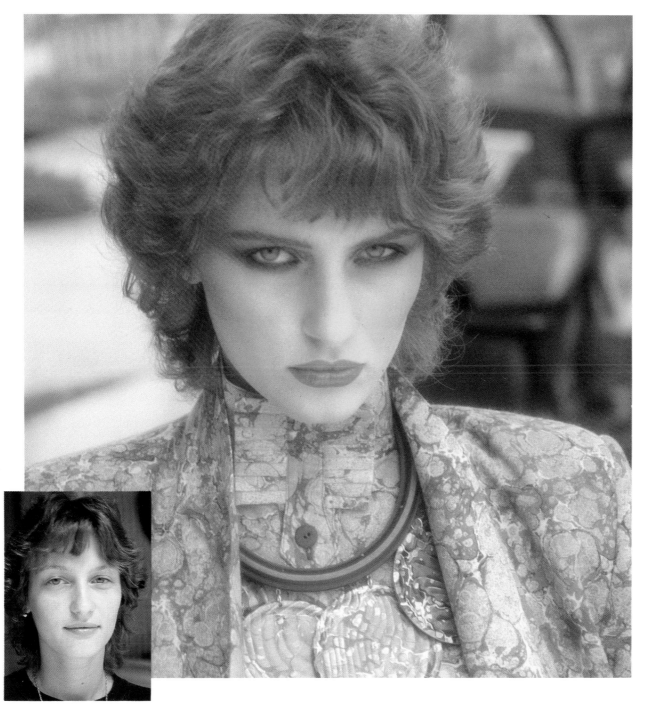

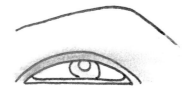

5. *Ivory powdered eye shadow* should then be applied under the eyebrow to highlight the browbone area.

6. Blend a *lightly frosted medium-gray powder shadow* out and upward at the corner of the eye, starting on the black pencil shading.

7. *Black eyeliner* is next applied at the base of the top lashes. Extend the line slightly beyond the outer corner of the eyes to lengthen them.

4

5

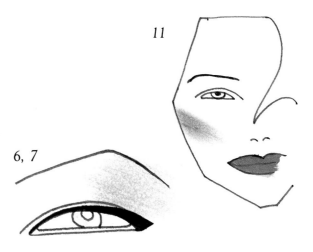

8. Use a *medium taupe pencil* to darken the eyebrows, as a stronger frame for this very strong eye.

9. Apply *black mascara* heavily to both top and bottom lashes.

10. Line inside the lower rim of the bottom lashes with a *black kohl pencil.*

11. Apply a *tawny powder blusher* low on the cheekbones.

12. Outline the already well-defined lips with a *bright red pencil.*

13. Use a lipbrush to apply *bright red lipstick.*

ruth

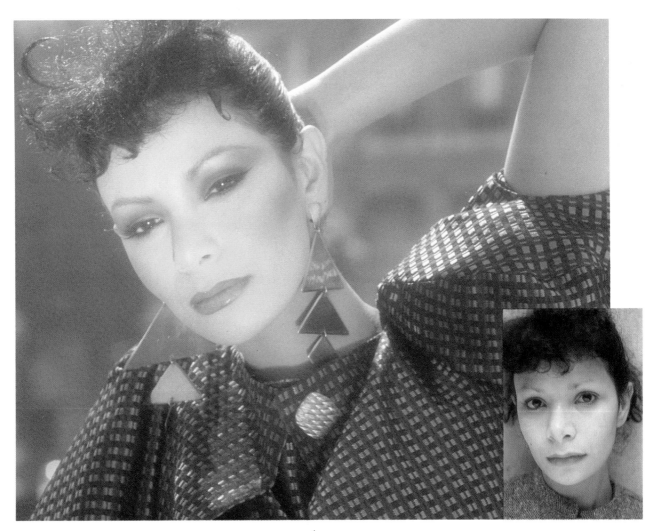

To modify:: The small eyes
The large mouth
To accentuate: Ruth's exotic facial structure and coloring

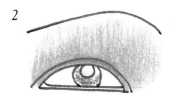

1. Use *beige foundation* on the face and eyelids.

2. Apply *bright red cream eye shadow* as close as possible to the base of the top lashes, then blend outward toward the end of the eyebrow.

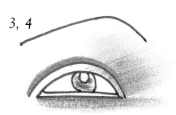

3. Use a *reddish-brown pencil* on the red shadow to darken the outer corner of the upper eyes, and in the socket crease from the inner corner next to the nose.

4. Apply a *dark green pencil* lightly at the base of the bottom lashes, blending slightly down and out.

5. Dust the entire face with a *transparent powder*, taking special care on the eyelids and under the eyes.

6. With a *taupe pencil* mixed with a little black, use short, fine strokes to draw in the eyebrows.

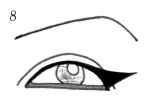

7. Blend a *frosted cream-colored highlighting powder* into the browbone under the eyebrow, covering a little of the red shadow.

8. Apply *black eyeliner* at the base of the top lashes, narrow at first, then becoming thicker, and extending out and upward, as shown.

9. Use a *dark green or black kohl pencil* inside the lower rim of the lashes.

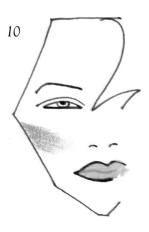

10. Apply a *golden-beige powder blusher* on the lower part of the cheekbones.

11. Outline the lips with a *light brown pencil*, taking care to draw just inside the natural line. Darken the corners of the mouth and blend well.

12. Color lips with a *beige lipstick*, beginning on the fullest part and overlapping the brown, though not completely covering it.

noriko

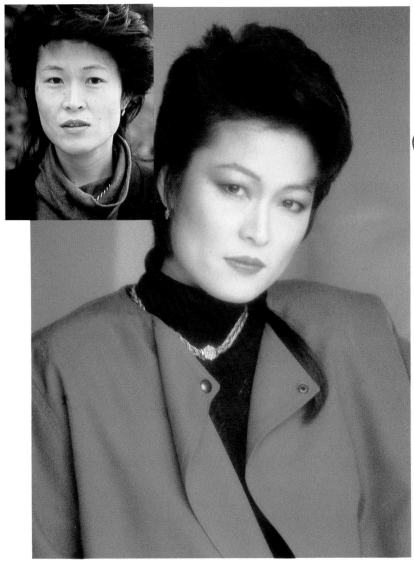

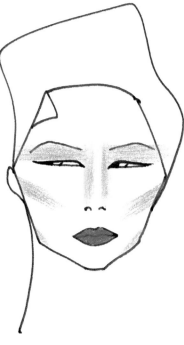

Aim: To adapt Aries makeup to an Oriental face

To enlarge the eyes and add dimension to the face

To emphasize the "businesswoman" image of Aries

Noriko's makeup is the same as Lilo's, with a slight difference at the eyes, since the Oriental eye has a fold rather than an

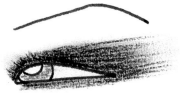

eye socket. The entire lid—that is, the epicanthic fold that extends almost to the base of the lashes—should be darkened with a black kohl pencil, and the shading well blended. Step 4 (the taupe eye shadow) should be eliminated, as should Step 7. Liner on the inside lower rim of the Oriental eye would close up the eye too much. To add dimension to the face, a brown matte contouring powder should be applied lightly and well blended on the inner part of the eyelid, down the sides of the nose, and under the cheek and jawbones.

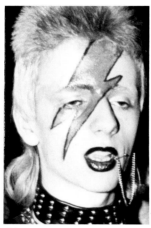

MARS-INSPIRED PUNK

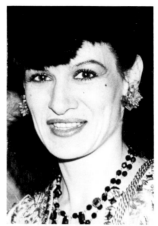

PALOMA PICASSO

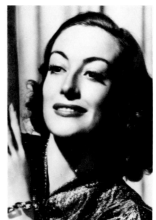

JOAN CRAWFORD

The ancient Greeks used cosmetics liberally in theatrical performances and religious rituals, where color was used to symbolize character. While respectable Greek women used little if any cosmetics, courtesans and men attending festive banquets were quite heavily made up. They whitened their faces and necks and colored their cheekbones and lips with a rust color made from oxygenated lead. Their eyelashes were thickened with a mixture of egg white, *noir de fumée* (a fine soot used as a pigment), and a primitive glue. They plucked their eyebrows completely and redrew them, and emphasized their nipples with red ocher. Apparently this was all done rather crudely, for they were a frequent target of many Greek satirists. These courtesans and men were the strong contemporary personalities of ancient Greece, much like the English male pop singers of today, who wear makeup as freely as female singers. Their aggressive Mars-inspired punk makeup is likewise governed by Aries.

Proving that even astrological history repeats itself, George Cukor once compared the extraordinarily sculptured face of Aries actress Joan Crawford to the finely chiseled mask of a fifth-century Grecian goddess. Ms. Crawford is probably the best example of the Aries woman's attitude toward fashion, as she believed that an intelligent woman is never a slave to fads. She loved earrings for the way they flatter and emphasize a woman's eyes, and bright clothing, but her makeup was always of neutral Aries tones. In the twenties, Ms. Crawford uncharacteristically attempted a style incompatible with her looks: her wide mouth was tortured into a tiny Cupid's bow. Later she emphasized her mouth and her large eyes (unusual for an Aries). She tweezed and penciled her eyebrows into dramatic arches, applied white pencil inside the rim of her lower lids, and always wore false eyelashes, which she ordered by the gross. By the 1950s, her beautiful thick eyebrows were natural once more.

The facial structure of Italian film star Claudia Cardinale is also representative of Aries. Her cheekbones are prominent and her eyes rather small. For a long time, she enlarged her eyes by darkening the eye area and applying eyeliner above the lashes, extending outward for nearly ⅛ of an inch. The lower inner rim and outer corner were lined with white, and false eyelashes applied to the base of the top lashes. By plucking and lifting the eye-

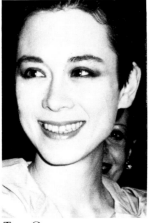

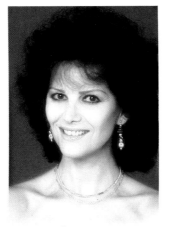

TINA CHOW   CLAUDIA CARDINALE

 brows and lightening the area just beneath them, she created an illusion of space in the upper eyelid area. Finally, to keep attention focused on her eyes, Ms. Cardinale deemphasized her mouth by using a pale lipstick, lightly applied. Now she seems to obtain her more contemporary look by using makeup tricks similar to those illustrated in the first Aries makeover.

Oriental beauty Tina Chow does not like the idea of makeup being used as a crutch or mask. She feels quite confident without any makeup at all, but appreciates the effect it can have. While she never wears mascara, her favorite makeup trick for a time was the use of gray kohl inside the rim of her eyes to enhance their hazel color. Now bright red lipstick is a favorite. She wears it alone or with a black pencil emphasizing her eyes. Tina dislikes blusher. Instead, she accentuates her already pale, transparent skin with a violet face powder.

Paloma Picasso is another great lover of red lipstick. She uses it to enhance her large, beautifully shaped mouth, after darkening her eyes slightly and using lots of black mascara. Like Tina, Paloma keeps her stunning cheekbones free of blusher.

t a u r u s
a p r i l 21 – m a y 20

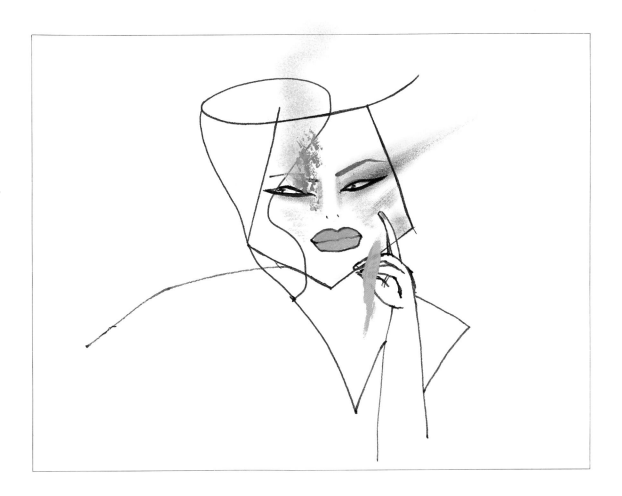

♉ Lucky Taurus! Her complexion is a perfect reflection of her character—strong, smooth, and, since she's ruled by Venus, extremely sensual. Photographs simply do not do her justice; her beauty lies in her "presence" as much as in her appearance. The first of the earth signs in nature's cycle, Taurus represents the land and is strongly based in the material. She is frequently found wearing no makeup, but because of her earthy, natural attractiveness, and since her skin is not prone to many problems, she is usually just as good-looking without it. Taurus, sure of her femininity, is unlike certain other signs which need makeup to boost their spirits; Cancer, for example, who uses makeup as part of her shell, to hide her sensitivity. Still, Taurus' artistic nature and love of beauty inspire a tremendous curiosity about makeup and its possibilities.

Taurus should use soft pink shades delicately to accentuate her innate sensuality, while dark yellow or mustard shades and natural greens and browns will emphasize her earthiness. She should also try metallic shades like copper and bronze, which are as softly flattering to her eyes as they are to her lips. Taurus' alternative to playing up the doe-like quality of her eyes is to make them stronger and more exotic by elongating them. This will widen that part of the face and add space to the sometimes close-set eyes. If Taurus wears her hair off her face, she should make her forehead lighter than the rest of her face by mixing a bit of white foundation with her usual color, or by dusting her brow with a white powder.

The often strong jaw can be deemphasized with a slightly darker foundation or taupe blusher *well blended* from under the cheekbones down to the jawbone. However, this trick should be used only at night. In daylight it can easily look like what it is: darker makeup on the lower part of the face. Knowledgeable Taureans minimize the lower part of the face by emphasizing the eyes instead. Blusher on the cheekbone itself should be a light pink shade. On the underside of the cheekbone (not in the hollow below it) a darker muted pink can be used, or russet or brown for a more earthy look. As earthier Taureans tend to have a rather thick neck, brown blusher can also be dusted down the sides of the neck (see sketch), with the most intense color at the top, just behind the jawbone. Those with thicker necks should

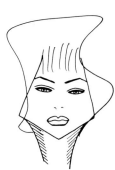

also avoid tight or heavy necklaces.

While her fellow earth signs, Capricorn and Virgo, must be selective and more light-handed with their bases, Taurus takes to almost any foundation well. Still, her natural glow should never be too heavily covered. Yellowish tints are the most attractive for her complexion, which has a beautiful touch of yellow itself. Pink shades of foundation will only drown this healthy, earthy skin tone.

Red is not the most flattering color for her lips, since it draws too much attention to the lower part of her face. Much better are the more neutral earth shades of russet, golden brown, or beige and almost all pale pinks except those that are frosted. Any of these harmonize beautifully with the coral and alabaster jewelry that is so lovely against her smooth skin. When Taurus wears her stone, the emerald, either in earrings or on a necklace, she would be wise to remember that these precious stones are almost all she needs to enhance her beauty. The most she would need in addition is black eye shadow or kohl pencil smudged around her eyes, very close to her lashes, a touch of brownish-pink blusher, and a muted lipstick—a natural but astonishingly glamorous look for the wild, natural beauty of the Taurus woman.

deborah

To modify: Close-set eyes
               Heavy jawbone
To accentuate: The natural earthy beauty
               of Taurus
               The color and quality of the
               skin

10, 11

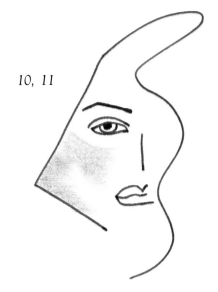

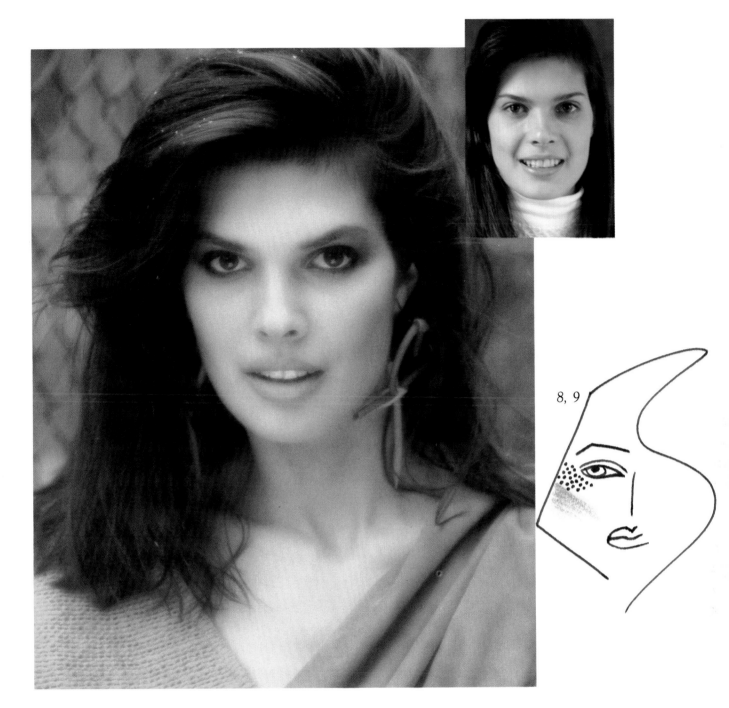

1. Apply a *lightweight, transparent beige foundation* to the whole of the face, including the eyelids. This will enhance the naturally beautiful complexion. Any pink-tinted foundations should be avoided, as they will destroy the ivory glow.

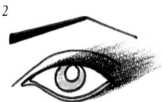

2. With a *black kohl pencil*, outline the outer part of the eye, applying it as close as possible to the lashes in the upper outer corner. Blend the pencil up and outward, leaving it dark next to the lashes.

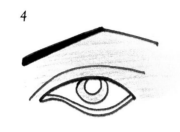

11

5, 6

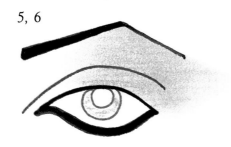

3. Powder the entire face, including the eyelids, with a *transparent face powder*.

4. Apply a light-to-medium *yellow-khaki eye shadow* to the entire eyelid. Use a little under the bottom lashes as well.

5. Blend a *dark khaki powder eye shadow* over the black pencil, taking it out and up into the lighter khaki shading.

6. Apply a *black kohl pencil* inside the lower rim of the eyes. This will make the eyes more almond-shaped.

7. Apply *black mascara* to both upper and lower lashes. Black mascara can harden the look of the other earth signs, Virgo and Capricorn, but Taurus' lashes are usually thick and dark,

and her soft, sensual features not easily hardened.

8. Dust a *translucent highlighter* or white powder lightly on top of the cheekbones. This will accentuate this part of the face, drawing attention away from the jawbone.

9. Blend a *light yellowish-brown matte powder blusher* under the cheekbones, to sculpt the face by emphasizing the bone structure.

10. Very delicately, shade the jawbone with this same powder. Transparent powder can be used to blend the blusher.

11. Blend a *light russet blusher* from the brown blusher over the cheekbones into the center of the cheeks, as shown in the sketch.

12. Do not line the lips, unless you want to draw more attention to them. Use a *light beige-colored lipstick*, following the naturally well-defined shape of the lips.

geri

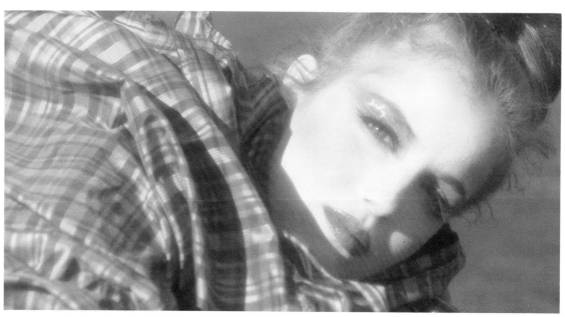

To modify: The heavy jawbone
To accentuate: The Venus-influenced sensuality of Taurus

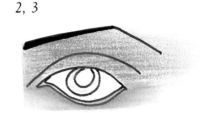

2, 3

1. Apply a *pale foundation* over the face and eyelids. It can be two shades lighter than the natural skin tone.

2. *Fuchsia powder eye shadow* or theatrical greasepaint should then be spread over the entire eyelid. Blend well into the foundation.

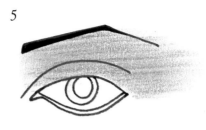

5

3. Color the base of the bottom lashes with a *russet pencil*. Blend well.

4. Dust the entire face, including eyelids and under-eye area, with a *transparent powder*.

5. Using a well-sharpened *soft gold pencil*, make uneven lines and shapes on the eyelid, as shown in the sketch.

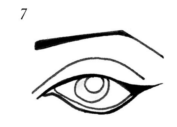

7

6. Accentuate the brightness of the gold by going over the lines with a *gold or bronze powder eye shadow*, applied with a very fine, wet brush.

7. Line the upper lid with a *black eyeliner*, narrow near the nose and thicker in the outer corner.

8. Apply *black mascara* to both top and bottom lashes.

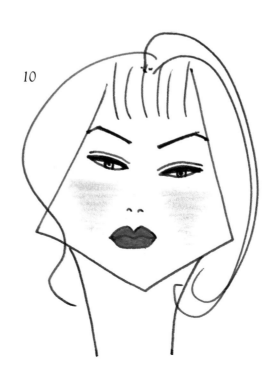

10

9. The third of a whole *false eyelash* should then be applied to the outer corner of the eye. To blend in with the natural lashes, it should first be shaped by cutting it irregularly, with the center shorter than the outer part.

10. Dust a *pale salmon powder blusher* on the center of the cheeks.

11. Use a *pale lilac face powder* to add an ethereal quality to the skin. Concentrate on the highest point of the cheekbones and avoid the jawbone.

12. Apply *burnt-orange lipstick* to the lips.

13

geri (2)

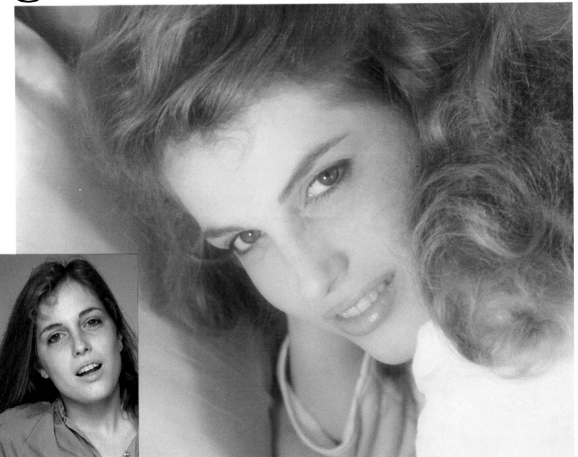

1. Apply a *pale ivory foundation* to the entire face, including the eyelids.

2. Spread a *pale pink cream blusher* over both eyelids, around and under the outer corner of the eye, and onto the cheekbones, blending it down slightly onto the cheeks. This will form a large halo around the outer part of the eyes.

3. Using a *very pale transparent powder* (perhaps transparent mixed with white), powder the entire face, especially the tinted areas. To keep this delicate effect, use no more color. (Option: to strengthen and dramatize this makeup, dust the already colored areas with a *shiny pale pink blusher or eye shadow.*)

4. Apply a *brown mascara* to accentuate the lashes and still maintain a soft effect.

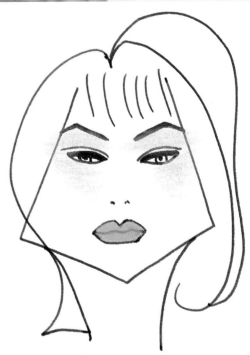

5. Line the lips with a *pale pink lip pencil*, taking care to blend the line well with a lipbrush.

6. Apply a *pale pink lipstick or lip gloss.*

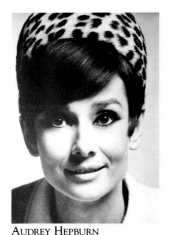
AUDREY HEPBURN

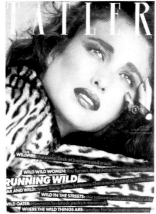
ANDIE MacDOWELL

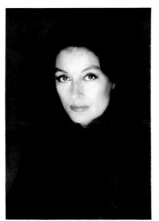
ANOUK AIMEE

Venus, goddess of beauty and love, influences the sign of Taurus and bestows on her the dark, exotic beauty characteristic of Egypt and Persia. It was in Egypt that eye makeup was perfected, for there the power of cosmetics was concentrated on the eyes, the instrument of strength for the Taurus woman. At the time of Nefertiti (long before Cleopatra popularized the heavy kohl lines drawn out to the middle of the forehead) eye makeup was refined. The brows were slightly narrowed at the end and curved gently inward toward the nose. A single kohl line defined the upper eyelid, which was shaded with a light pink made from crushed rose petals or a green powdered crystal derived from a silicate of copper. This pink shading was also used on the cheekbones. The inner part of the lid, the nostrils, and the earlobes were highlighted with a touch of light golden saffron, while the lips were left natural. Imperfections of the skin were often smoothed out with a light layer of henna, and the complexion was always well protected from the elements. Round black beauty marks were applied, and to emphasize the transparency of their skin, women accented the veins of their foreheads with a blue pencil.

Taurus beauty in its essence is also characterized by a wonderfully proportioned body, graceful movements, and physical magnetism, all of which combine to make many women of this sign top runway models. Alva Chin is a perfect example of this.

Actress-singer Cher is quite similar to Alva, with a longer, narrower face and smaller lips than most Taureans. Cher's large doe-like eyes are even more outstanding because of her narrower face, and although she adores makeup, she is extremely beautiful without it. It makes perfect sense that Cher's sign rules Egypt; she would be a perfect Egyptian princess with her coloring, her large eyes, and her strong features.

As Taurus is the sign of the bull, many Taureans have facial features similar to the bull. This is by no means a drawback! One of the best examples is Audrey Hepburn, with her enormous, limpid eyes. In the past, Ms. Hepburn emphasized their doe-like quality by encircling them with a soft black pencil, applying a white pencil inside the lower rim, and using black mascara lavishly on the upper and lower lashes. Her small forehead was astutely balanced with wispy bangs, and her strong, perfectly

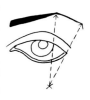

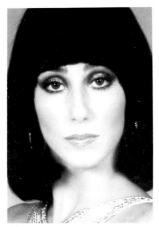
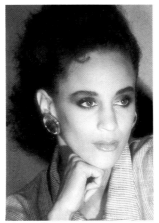

CHER   ALVA CHIN

arched eyebrows are also typically Taurean. Her sensual lips were minimized with a light lipstick.

French film actress Anouk Aimee is another typical Taurus, and the ideal beauty of celebrated designer Karl Lagerfeld. Her face, he says, is "classical, timeless, and discreet"—a face beyond fashion. It's no surprise that Karl prefers "earthy" colors, perfect for Taurus.

Photographic model Andie MacDowell was chosen by Calvin Klein (Scorpio) to represent his jeans. For this campaign her Taurean sensuality was emphasized. Note her full, sensual lips and thick dark (Taurean) hair. Andie is also a favorite of film director Hugh Hudson, who found her

qualities of shyness and vulnerability, magnified by her smoldering beauty, perfect for the role of Jane in his film *Greystoke: The Legend of Tarzan*. Andie's makeup for the film was extremely simple. A little bit of concealer was applied under the eyes, and her already pale skin was dusted with a light, transparent powder. She wore no mascara, although some brown color was applied to her lower lashes to darken them slightly. Amber blusher was used on her cheeks, but she bit her lips and pinched her cheeks frequently to make natural color come to them. When Andie does her own makeup, she wears dark brown eye shadow, or black eyeliner when in a more dramatic mood.

g e m i n i
m a y 21 – j u n e 20

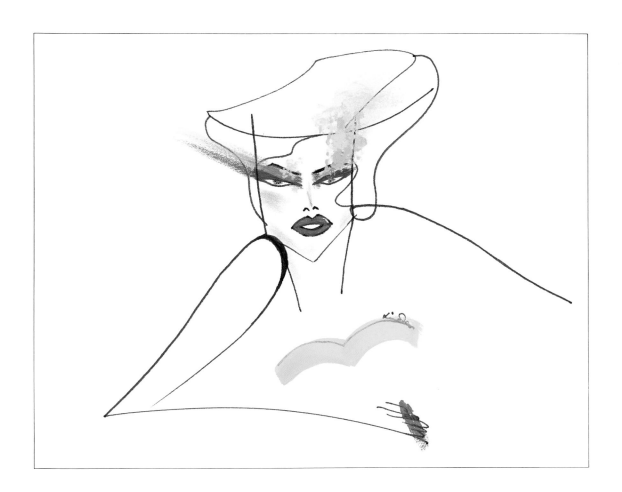

Ⅱ The extremely pretty, lively, and intelligent-looking Gemini woman has the most beautiful profile in the zodiac. She has elegantly sculptured features: a well-formed nose that can be either dainty or long and straight; full lips, clearly defined and well colored; and almond-shaped eyes that tend to slant upward. Her face is either long, nicely balanced and rectangular, or triangular because of prominent cheekbones. Although it's usually hidden by her hair, Gemini's identifying feature is her forehead. There is always something unusual about the

Gemini brow, whether it's a perfect widow's peak such as that of Brooke Shields, or a distinctly odd shape. The Gemini woman also has a clear, glowing complexion that tans easily and retains its color for a long time. Hers is a timeless face; it changes little and never seems to wrinkle as she gets older.

With such versatile features, Gemini has quite a few options for choosing and applying makeup—and with her famous mercurial personality, she enjoys experimenting with all of them. Still, there are some basic guidelines to consider.

Very little foundation should be used on that perfect complexion. If there are dark circles under the eyes, a pale but warm-colored concealer or foundation can be used, followed by a translucent or golden powder to blend and smooth.

Those remarkable eyes should be accentuated. Dark eye shadow should be used sparingly under the eyes to emphasize the almond shape. Some delicate penciling is enough; then, additional light penciling at the base of the upper lashes is all Gemini will need for pretty definition within an overall natural look. For slightly more emphasis, she can use black, dark gray, or navy eyeliner at the base of the upper lashes, extending the line out and up to follow the tilt of the eyes. With lots of mascara, this is an easy, effective alternative to using eye shadows. The diversity of Gemini's nature, however, will probably lead her to experiment successfully with colors and unusual combinations. Bright blues, yellows, and reds—as well as violet with green, orange with violet—can all be worn by the chameleon-like Gemini. But for the most glamorous look, she should don a pair of aquamarine earrings and opt for dark, smoky eyes. Aquamarine is her stone: sparkling near, and with, her eyes, it creates an irresistible effect. The final step in tending to her eye makeup involves the eyebrows. Although they hardly ever need plucking, she should remember to brush them into shape to enhance their naturally graceful arch.

Very little blusher is needed with prominent cheekbones. It should always be applied last, to avoid any conflict in coloring or intensity. A lighter touch is needed if the eyes and lips are bright, in order to avoid a clown-like effect. Depending on the colors of her clothing and makeup, either beige, amber, or brown should be applied on the cheekbones themselves, to soften angles. For more drama, that same color can be used in the hollow of the cheeks, with a slightly lighter color on the cheekbones to emphasize their angularity.

Gemini looks most stunning with a clear, bright red lipstick. With those well-shaped lips, though, any color—matte, iridescent, or gloss—will be very flattering.

laure

To accentuate: The angular face
The oblique, almond-shaped eyes
The mysterious side of Gemini's nature

1. Apply a *very pale foundation* to the entire face.

2. With a *blue-violet pencil*, color the up-

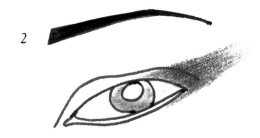

per corners of the outer eyes, and bring the color slightly under the eye. Blend gently.

18

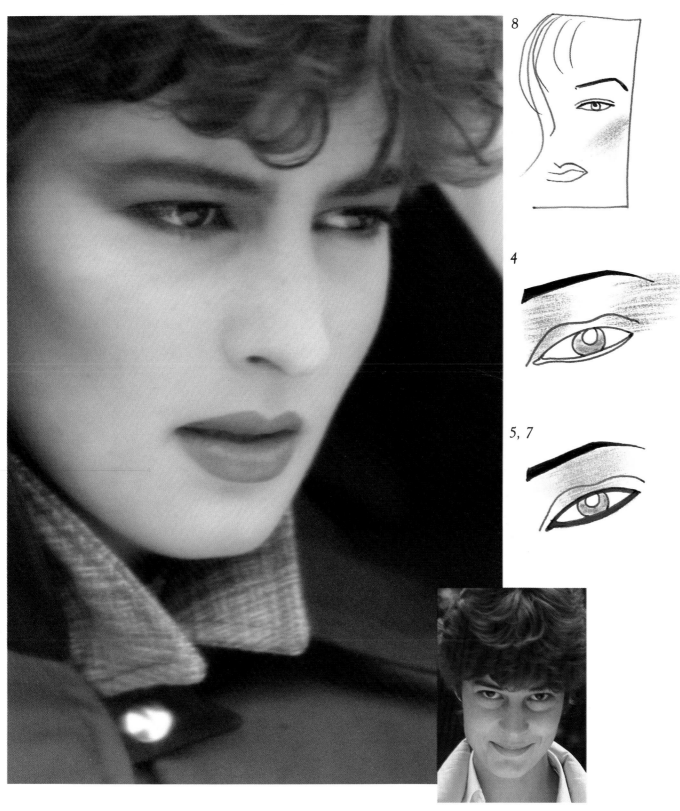

8

4

5, 7

3. Apply *transparent powder* over the entire face, including the eyelids.

4. Blend a *violet matte powder eye shadow* from the top lashes upward and over the pencil, feathering past the eyebrows. Blend the same shadow in the inner corners of the eyes, next to the nose, upward to the eyebrow.

5. Blend a *yellow-green powder eye shadow* from the eyelashes in the center of the eye up to the eyebrows, and into the violet shadow.

6. Apply *black mascara* to upper and lower lashes.

19

7. Apply a *violet-colored kohl pencil* inside the upper and lower rims of the eyes.

8. Blend a *brown shade of powder blusher* on the lower part of the cheekbone.

9. Apply a *bright red lipstick*, following the perfect line of the lips.

veronica

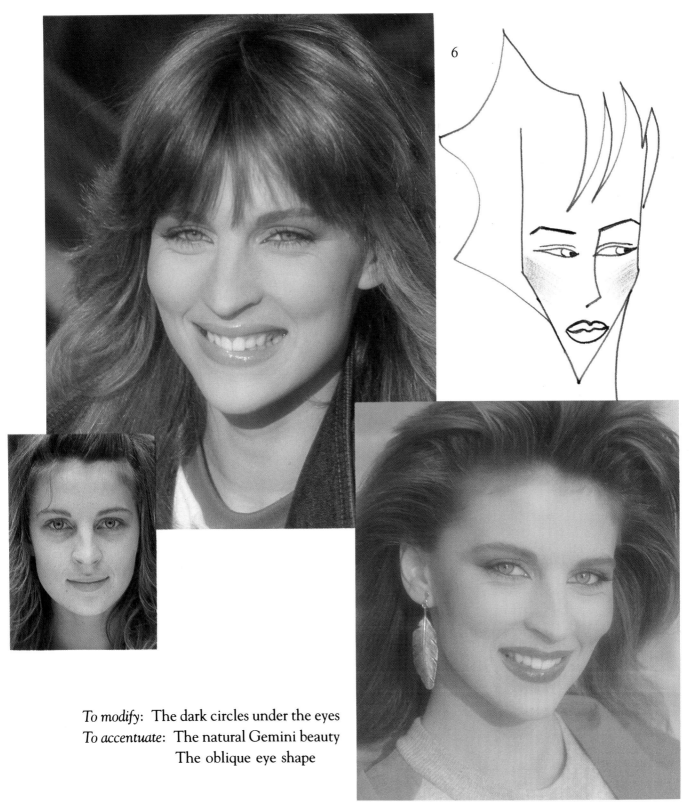

6

To modify: The dark circles under the eyes
To accentuate: The natural Gemini beauty
The oblique eye shape

1. Apply a *medium beige foundation* to the entire face.

2. Apply a *lighter beige under-eye concealer* and blend into the foundation.

3. Apply a *medium blue-green pencil* delicately in the outer corner of the eye, at the base of the upper and lower lashes, and in the outer part of the eye socket.

4. Powder the face and eyelids with a *transparent powder.*

5. Apply a *mustardy-beige matte powder eye shadow* over the entire eyelid, including the already shaded part.

6. Apply an *amber-colored blusher* to the cheekbones.

7. Apply a *dark green kohl pencil* inside the lower rim of the eyes.

8. Apply *black mascara* to both top and bottom lashes.

9. Apply a *transparent lip gloss.*

3

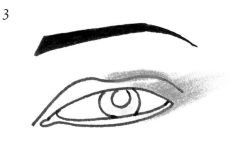

5, 7

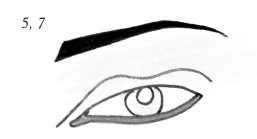

To achieve a more glamorous effect, as shown in the second picture of Veronica, add a bright red lipstick.

caroline

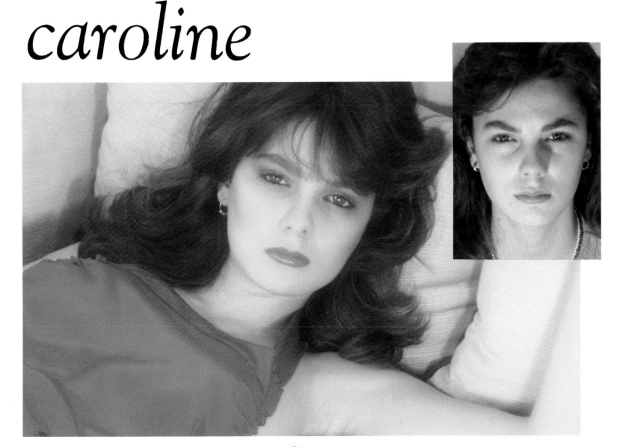

To modify: A rather wide nose

To accentuate: Gemini versatility, with an unusual mixture of colors

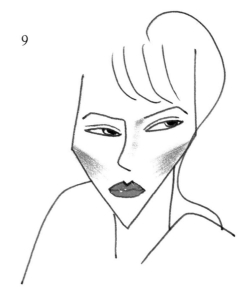

1. To set off the colors of the eye shadows, apply *foundation* in a slightly lighter shade than actual skin color.

2. Powder the entire face with a *transparent powder*.

3. Cover the eyelid completely with a *bright orange matte powder eye shadow*, blending it outward. Apply the same color lightly under the eyes.

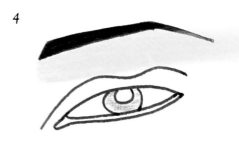

4. Blend a *bright yellow powder eye shadow* under the eyebrow over the eyebrow bone.

5. Blend a *bright pink powder eye shadow* in the outer upper corner of the eyes next to the lashes.

6. Apply *black mascara* to both top and bottom lashes.

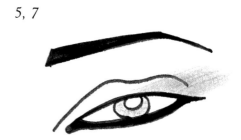

7. Apply *black kohl pencil* inside the lower rim of the eyes. This intensifies their expression by accentuating their shape.

8. Blend *lilac powder* lightly onto the cheekbones.

9. Blend a *medium-brown matte powder blusher* under the cheekbones and from the beginning of the eyebrows down the sides of the nose to the tip.

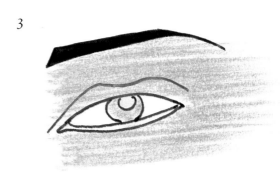

10. Outline the lips with a *red lip pencil*.

11. Fill in the lips with a *bright red lipstick*.

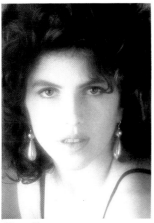

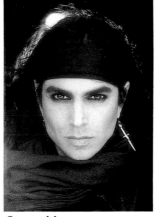

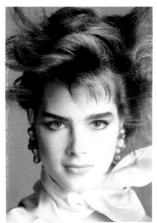

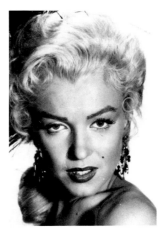

CLIO GOLDSMITH   STEVEN MEISEL   BROOKE SHIELDS   MARILYN MONROE

John Sahag (Capricorn) loves makeup of all kinds and colors on a woman—even the most outrageous—as long as it is in harmony with her looks and style. It is overall beauty that attracts him most, one that is enhanced by sensitivity, honesty, and self-confidence. He finds Brooke Shields a perfect example, and notes that her wonderfully pure beauty is also marked by what he calls "an extraordinary avant-garde sensuality." Together, they produce in Brooke the epitome of the modern, confident Gemini beauty.

Although her perfectly chiseled face is stunning without any cosmetics at all, Brooke loves makeup and is most comfortable with a touch of amber-colored blusher and the pale frosted lipsticks that she adores. Her personal tastes change with the changing fashions, and she enjoys experimenting with many effects. The pinks and purples that were her favorite colors have been replaced by browns, bronzes, and greens—and in true Gemini style, she looks gorgeous in any of these hues.

The fashion in Marilyn Monroe's era was softer and more sensual, and she arranged her hairstyle and applied her makeup to lessen the angularity of her face. Although her hair was dyed blond, she left her eyebrows dark—and at times even darkened them further. It was an original effect, and resulted in wonderfully provocative eyes when combined with her equally original eye makeup. Marilyn lightened her entire eyelid with a pale, frosty color, and darkened the eye socket slightly. Then, instead of applying her eyeliner in a gradually widening line from the inner to the outer corners of her eyes, she drew the line a millimeter thicker in the beginning and over the iris, then narrowed it, drawing it up and out. A few false eyelashes were added in the corners.

Marilyn's pale, creamy complexion was most often free of blusher, although when her makeup was shinier, she applied a touch of color directly onto her cheekbones (again, softening those angles). Her final touch was the bright red lipstick she loved, which emphasized perfectly her beautiful Gemini smile and teeth. The full, pouty shape of her lips can be achieved with a red pencil. Smooth out the heart of the lips as shown, then lift the corners of the upper lip. Outline the upper lip with a gentle arc, with the highest point at the midpoint. The outline of the lower lip should curve downward symmetrically with the curve of the upper lip—go down *under*

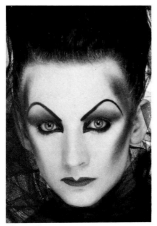

BOY GEORGE

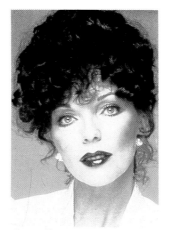

JOAN COLLINS

the lip line in the center.

Actress Clio Goldsmith never wears foundation on her flawless, vibrant Gemini complexion. She plays up the beauty of her sign with mascara, a touch of brown at the base of her lashes, and a muted natural shade of lipstick or lip gloss.

Joan Collins, on the other hand, enjoys emphasizing the more glamorous side of her nature. She accentuates her high cheekbones with shading below the bone and an earthy color on the cheekbone itself. She is a typical Gemini not only in her looks but in her love of purple eye shadows and fuchsia lipsticks as well. Her sign's other colors, such as green and yellow, would also look wonderful on her, but brown would be too tame for her dynamic beauty.

It is interesting to note, in view of the makeup-loving nature of this sign, that even Gemini men enjoy the versatility and whimsy that cosmetics afford them. Singer Boy George has looks typical of his sign: almond-shaped eyes, beautiful eyebrows, and an extremely unusual forehead. He always wears foundation for a matte effect. The violets, yellows, and pinks that were once his favorite colors have recently given way to more subdued shades; his favorites

of late seem to be grays worn with orange-red lipstick. He reshapes his eyebrows completely—four of the many shapes he uses are pictured. To obtain his eye makeup effect, you may lengthen the eyes with a pencil in the outer corner, blending it up and outward. He also uses black kohl inside the lower rim of the eyes and a little at the base of the upper and lower lashes. This is followed with black mascara. It is also important to outline the lips with a red pencil, as he emphasizes or sometimes reshapes his mouth completely when making up.

Steven Meisel, renowned fashion photographer, changes his look constantly, in true mercurial Gemini style, and is a great promoter of avant-garde makeup. Sometimes, like Boy George, he draws his eyebrows straight up and out from the apex. At other times, he makes them square in shape—or even makes them into one brow, as shown. He has sported both white and tanned complexions with red lips, but his eye makeup is generally consistent: dark and smoky, with kohl inside the lower rim and dark shading right up to the eyebrows. He also uses shading to accentuate the beautiful shape of his Gemini face.

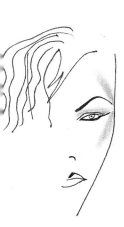

cancer

june 21 – july 22

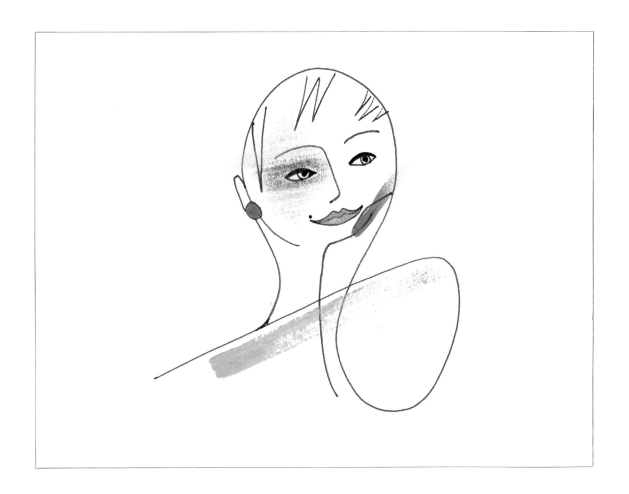

The Cancer woman is like the moon that rules her: constant only in her changeability. Her beauty is a concentration of many lunar qualities—dreaminess and mutability are the most compelling—and she certainly knows how to make the most of her assets. However, the sensitive moon child easily becomes depressed and self-pitying and then is apt to be rather lazy about her appearance. She must be cajoled and flattered into emerging from her shell and confidently displaying her Cancerian spirit—whether it's characterized by a re-fined, exquisite taste or an intriguing, original style.

While her appearance and makeup reflect her instinct for what suits her best, they are not always conventional (especially if she is accentuating her special lunar madness) and can leave her open to negative reaction. If she so wishes, she can play it safe by emphasizing her soft lunar mystery instead. By gently blending her moon colors of palest gold, pale greens, opalescent blues, and iridescent hues of lilac and purple around her eyes, she'll create a shimmering halo of color to en-

25

hance her dreamy expression. Violet or dark blue pencils applied inside the lower rim of the eyes will emphasize the color of the iris as well as that special faraway look. All harsh lines should be avoided, in her blusher and lip pencil as well as her eye shadow and liner.

Cancer's expressive, serene face has a tendency to allergies and burns easily in the sun. She must take rigorous care of her complexion, especially as it is affected greatly by her state of mind. To protect it in the harsh city environment, the palest of creamy foundations—even an iridescent one—should be used. The beauty of her radiant, lunar white skin can then be enhanced with a dusting of the finest, palest gold or silver iridescent powder. If her rising sign is Capricorn or Virgo, she may have a somewhat sluggish complexion. In this case, a pale foundation is necessary for appearance as well as protection.

It's unnecessary to encourage the Cancer woman to experiment. She will follow her feelings and moods, to project or protect her personality. Her distinctive style will eventually comprise many different looks, as befits her changeable nature. There are, however, physiognomic differences among Cancer women which call for slight variations in their makeup, regardless of the style they choose.

The "full-moon" type is the one most people think of when they picture the Cancer woman. She has a large skull, overhanging brow, and pronounced jaw, with small, round, wide-set eyes and a short, slightly wide nose. She may have a real "baby face"—full and round, with a narrow forehead. Usually this type has fine blond hair as well. The lips have a narrow bow shape, like that fashionable in the twenties—often with a beauty mark on or overlapping them. The "half-moon" Cancer is more sensual and frequently more Mediterranean-looking. Her face is much narrower, her eyes—most often brown— more closely set, her nose is a little longer and turns down slightly, and her lips are fuller. The baby-faced Cancer, while not needing as great an intensity of color around her eyes as the half-moon type, does require quite a lot of color to enlarge her eyes.

Pale silvery shades of salmon-pink lipstick are best for the full-moon Cancer's ethereal looks, but all violets, clear pinks, and even orange lipsticks would be flattering to the half-moon Cancer, whose full lips need no enlarging (although she will probably do this, nonetheless).

Transparent or milky stones such as the opal, moonstone, pearls, and crystal are ruled by the moon and are therefore governed by Cancer. They blend perfectly with any makeup she might choose—from the most classic to the most imaginative— and complement wonderfully her smooth, shimmery complexion and her luminous otherworldly beauty.

emilie

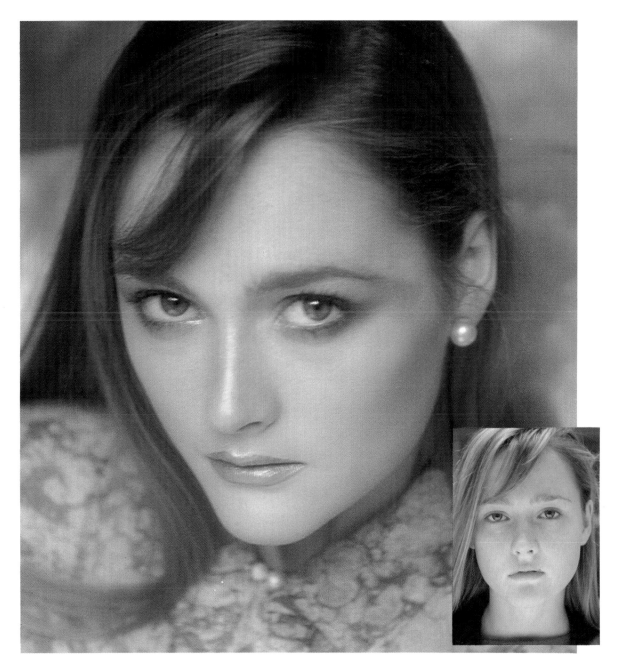

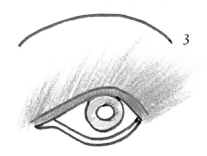

To modify: The redness in the cheeks
The small, wide-set eyes and flat eyelids
The broad forehead
The heavy, square jaw

To accentuate: The smooth, luminous skin
The golden gleam in the eyes

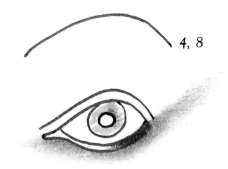

1. Apply a *green tinted moisturizer*.

2. With this type of skin, no foundation would be necessary for a natural makeup in neutral tones. As this makeup is quite colorful, however, and since we are modifying the shape of the face, a *light shade of foundation* with good coverage is necessary.

3. A *very dark green pencil* should then be applied quite heavily, as close as possible to the base of the top lashes. Blend up and outward, leaving the color heavier next to the lashes.

4. Apply a *violet pencil* to the base of the bottom lashes, blending down and slightly inward to the nose, then out and upward to join the green at the outer corner.

5. Dust the entire face, including the eyelids and under-eye area, with a *transparent powder*.

6. Blend a *pale gold powder eye shadow* from the eyebrow bone down across the lid, going lightly over the green. Take this color from the eyebrow around to the top of the cheekbone to highlight this area.

7. Blend a little *grayish-brown matte powder blusher* or dark face powder from the inner eyebrows down the sides of the nose.

8. Apply a *dark purple kohl pencil* in the outer corner of the bottom rim of the eyes.

9. Brush the same blusher used in Step 7 around the forehead at the hairline and down onto the jawbone, making it slightly stronger under the cheekbone. Always blend inward, and avoid sharp lines and stops by mixing the blusher with a little natural face powder.

7, 9

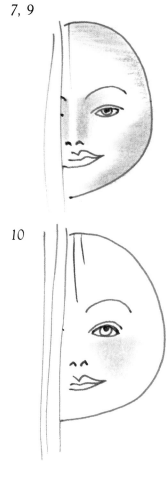

10

12

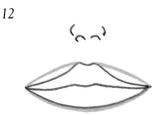

10. A *bluish-pink powder blusher* is then blended onto the cheeks, starting half on the darker brown shading and half on the golden highlighter on the cheekbones.

11. Dust the forehead, the center of the nose, the chin, and the heart of the lips with a *gold highlighting powder*.

12. Outline the lips, slightly outside their natural line, with a *light peach-colored pencil*.

13. Apply a *pale silvery-peach lipstick*.

14. Add a touch of *gold highlighter* to the center of the bottom lip.

jody

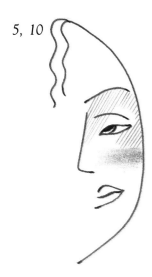

5, 10

3

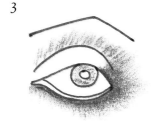

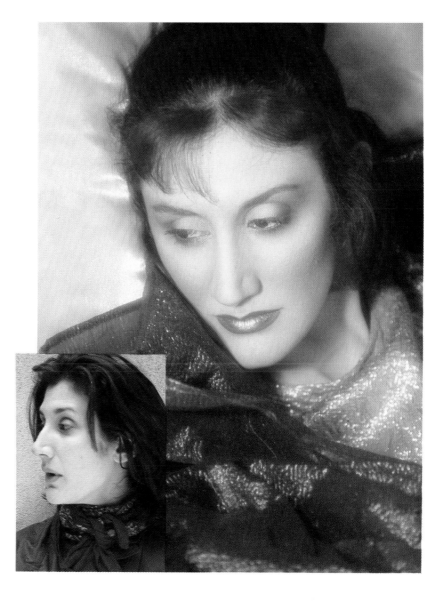

To modify: The small, deep, close-set eyes
 The rather long face
To accentuate: The exotic cheekbones
 The beautiful ivory skin

1. Apply a *yellow cream or ivory foundation* to the entire face and eyelids. Avoid all pink shades on this skin tone.

2. With a *very pale under-eye cream*, lighten the inner corners of the eyes, both above and beneath the eyes, and the mobile part of the lids.

3. With a *violet pencil*, color from the deepest part of the eye, blending onto the eyebrow bone, then around and under the eye at the base of the bot-

tom lashes. Keep the color very intense next to the lashes and gradually lighten it as you blend out and down.

4. Apply a little of this same violet in the outer corner of the upper lashes, to darken and space the eyes.

5. Apply a *pale gold powder* onto the already lightened part of the eyelid and around the violet part onto the cheekbone. Blend it slightly into the violet.

6. Apply a *pale frosted turquoise powder* to the mobile part of the eyelid already covered with the gold.

7. Apply *black mascara* to both top and bottom lashes.

8. Line inside the lower rim of the eyes with a *deep violet kohl pencil.*

9. If the eyebrows are sparse, it is very important that they be slightly thickened and arched with light, fluffy strokes of a *grayish-brown pencil* to frame the eyes well.

10. The length of the face is broken by applying a *brownish powder blusher* just under the cheekbone. Blend it straight across the face toward the nose.

11. A little *salmon-pink powder blusher* should then be applied in the center of the cheeks to give more fullness.

12. Use a *dark bluish-red pencil* to slightly enlarge the natural lip line.

13. Apply with a lipbrush a *pinkish-violet lipstick.*

14. To give more shape to the lips, apply a touch of *pale gold highlighter* to the center of the upper and lower lips.

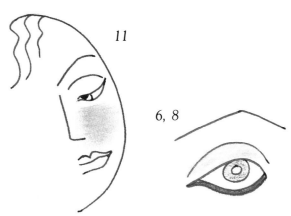

melodie

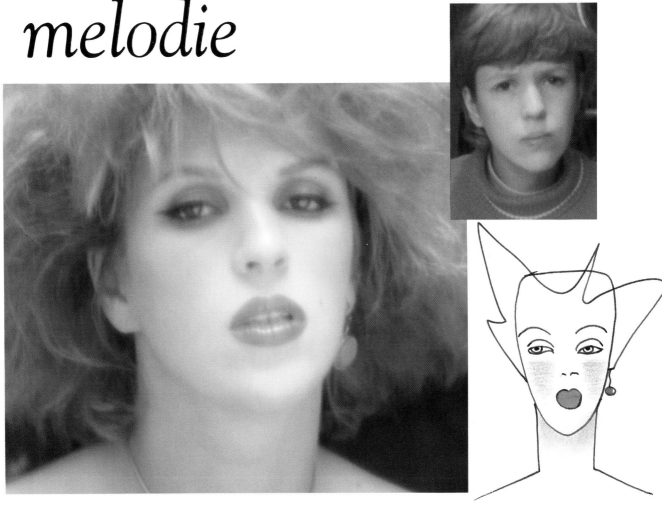

To modify: The poorly defined jawbone
          The rather wide neck
To accentuate: Cancerian sensuality

1. Apply an *ivory foundation* to the entire face.

2. Lightly powder the entire face with a *pale transparent powder.*

3. To the upper lid apply a *green iridescent powder eye shadow*, blending it slightly

outward. Blend a little of the same eye shadow under the eye.

4. Draw a line of *black eyeliner*, starting fine in the inner corner and becoming thicker toward the outside. Extend the line past the outer corner.

5. A *vivid salmon-pink lipstick* should be taken well to the outer edge of the lips.

6. Apply a *powder blusher* in a harmonizing shade. To avoid lengthening the face, apply it low on the cheekbone and take the color straight across the face from the outer edge, rounding the color more in the center as shown.

7. Apply *black mascara* to upper and lower lashes.

8. Just under the jawbone, apply a *medium-brown blusher*. Blend down onto the neck.

Cancer is a sensitive, emotional, and, above all, nurturing sign. It rules closely knit family groups and tribes and is particularly close to the vibrations of black African peoples. In a typically Cancerian way, makeup is used for decorative purposes rather than as a sign of social status. The pygmies of Central Africa, the Xhosa of South Africa, and the Masai all use face and body makeup, but none have perfected it to the extent of the Nuba of Kau in the Sudan. Makeup is their medium of artistic expression, and they regard their bodies as the consummation of their art. Unless they are working in the fields, the marriageable male Nubas paint and adorn themselves daily—sometimes even changing "masks" again in the course of the day. Using paints derived from charcoal, shells, and stones, they adeptly accentuate their best features and conceal or direct attention away from their blemishes. They have fantastic imagination and a strong feeling for graphic design: when they paint the two halves of their faces asymmetrically, the final effect is nonetheless harmonious, as they have an extraordinary talent for using seemingly incongruous lines and shapes to create balance. These tendencies—the constant changing of styles and the ability to rec-

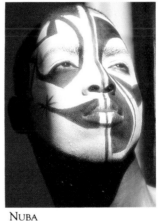 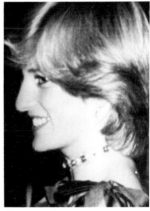

NUBA   PRINCESS DIANA

oncile seemingly "off-balance" designs—are quintessentially Cancerian. The Nuba females are equally enthusiastic about adorning their bodies. From the age of approximately four years, they anoint themselves with oil and pigments ranging from yellow to red. Each clan wears a special shade, unless, of course, it's unflattering to a particular girl's skin. In this case, she is allowed to wear another shade.

Princess Diana has a perfect Cancerian profile (note the nose and chin), fine eyebrows, and rather small eyes. Her satin-smooth complexion always has a slight glow and is never covered with much powder, and she has a natural redness to her cheeks. Princess Diana adapts her makeup to the occasion: during the day it is discreet, with a pale lipstick or lip gloss, a light shadow on the eyelid, and light brown

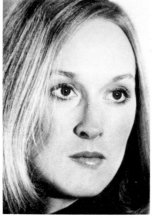

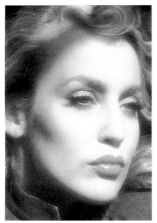

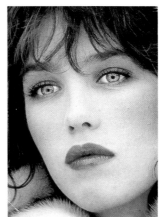

MERYL STREEP   JERRY HALL   ISABELLE ADJANI

in the crease and blended slightly outward. She always wears kohl—usually blue, but sometimes black—inside the lower rim of the lashes, and lots of mascara. Occasionally she lines the outer edge of the base of her upper lashes for further definition. Her blusher is a subtle tawny or pink. For more formal occasions, she seems to favor the sparkling gold so flattering to her sign. She wears it on the mobile part of her eyelid, and will sometimes apply it to her cheekbones for a glittery effect.

Designer Thierry Mugler (Sagittarius) likes makeup that reveals one's personality. He feels that the beauty of a woman lies in her "aura"—a certain fragility and a feeling of softness, but with a sparkling humor enlivening it. These are all Cancerian qualities, so it is little wonder that Jerry Hall and Meryl Streep are two of his favorite beauties.

Sexy, beautiful Jerry Hall is a great lover of makeup. Although she does not have the round face typical of many Cancers, without makeup Jerry has a very definite baby face. Like most women of her sign, however, she is rarely seen without makeup. During the day, Jerry wears base,

powder, a pink-tinted rust eye shadow, and lots of mascara. Her blusher and lipstick are coordinated. In the evening, she enjoys sparkling eye shadows and lip colors and dramatically lines the base of her upper and lower lashes with black eyeliner pencil. After smudging the liner with her finger, she applies false eyelashes to the base of her upper lashes to lengthen and strengthen them.

The beauty of Meryl Streep is dizzyingly mutable, as befits her sign. Her small, amused blue-green eyes seem to change whenever she changes clothing, or roles. She has qualities of both types of Cancer—the pale, luminous skin of the full-moon type and the narrow face and longer nose of the half-moon. Although she wears no makeup on an everyday basis, she will wear whatever seems right for her roles.

Dazzling blue eyes and a naturally superb complexion are the outstanding features of the dreamy, expressive French film star Isabelle Adjani. Like Meryl Streep, she enjoys wearing a variety of makeup for her various roles, and her protean nature allows her to portray a wide range of qualities through her appearance.

l e o
j u l y 2 3 – a u g u s t 2 1

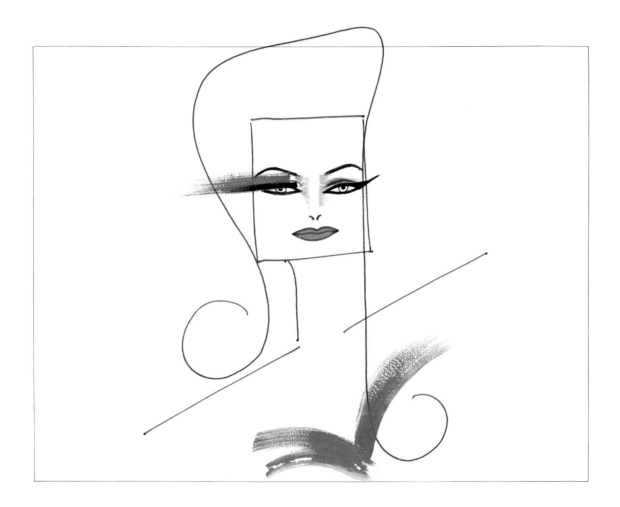

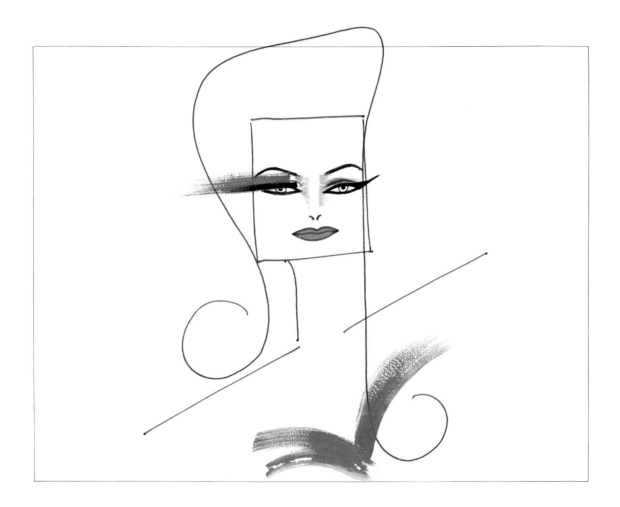 The strong radiant beauty of the Lioness stems from the combination of her love for life and her regal bearing. The beautiful expression in her eyes can be soft and calm one minute, then sparkling and lively when her enthusiasm overwhelms her contentment. Although Leo has a rectangular face with a wide, flat forehead, it is softer and wider than the rectangular Gemini face. She has well-shaped features—a regal nose and a rather small mouth, with the lower lip fuller than the upper lip—but her best assets are beautiful cheekbones and round, upturned eyes.

Despite her artistic inclinations, the Leo woman does not have an innate talent for using makeup to her advantage. The shape of her eyes makes them difficult to make up, so she can be more attractive without, rather than with, incorrectly applied cosmetics. Furthermore, Leo is frequently unable to see herself objectively. For this reason, she needs to practice applying makeup and should seek advice and feedback from her friends. Although Leo loves the limelight, she has a tendency to underplay her regality and sophistication, as if their physical manifestation were unimportant or cause for embarrassment. Here again her friends can be most helpful, by giving her the warmth and encouragement she needs to be at her best. Above all, Leo should remember that she is at her most beautiful, and most in harmony with herself, when her extravagant, luxurious nature is emphasized.

This does not mean that a natural makeup is inappropriate for her. On the contrary, while the bright colors she loves so much are suitable for her clothing, I advise neutral tones for her eyes—especially elegant shades of gray or brown. If her eyes are blue, a touch of the blue closest to her eye color can be combined with gray or brown. She should also remember to enhance her characteristic subtle elegance by lightening the browbone with a silvery-gray or grayish-white highlight. With a somewhat underplayed eye makeup, the ardent nature of this fire sign can be emphasized instead with the bright red and ruby lipsticks which are most flattering for her, or with Leo-governed ruby jewelry. Since Leo's upper lip is often asymmetrical, it is advisable to line the lips before applying lipstick. If only a muted-pink lipstick is to be worn, pinkish-beige or natural pencil is best. Once Leo has discovered the best way to use these colors and feels comfortable applying them, she can lessen the intensity of her eye makeup and use only lip gloss when in a more relaxed, playful mood.

Special attention should be paid to the dry skin of fairer-haired Leos. Mild cleansers and a nightly nourishing cream will stabilize and strengthen the complexion. The brunette's skin is stronger and more even-textured than the ruddier blonde's. For her, a warmish beige foundation or even a golden tint would be best to lessen the pink. More Leo women color their hair a golden blond than women of any other sign; in such cases, they will need a foundation color that adds a golden warmth to their skin tone.

Leos love plenty of real jewelry. Gold, their metal, accentuates the warm glow of their skin, and lots of it—in oversized earrings or several gold necklaces, for example—will enhance the exoticism that is so much a part of the brunette's appeal. The more quietly regal blonde will find that sparkling diamonds are the perfect accompaniment to her luxurious, sophisticated beauty.

susan

To modify: The very round eyes
　　　　　The small upper lip
　　　　　The reddish tint to the nose
To accentuate: The beautiful prominent
　　　　　cheekbones
　　　　　The intensity of the eyes

1. To retain the transparency of this fine freckled skin, a little *very pale foundation* was applied only to the eyelids, the nose, the chin, and the under-eye area. This must be extremely well matched to the skin tone and well blended.

2. A little *concealer* was applied with a small brush to blemishes.

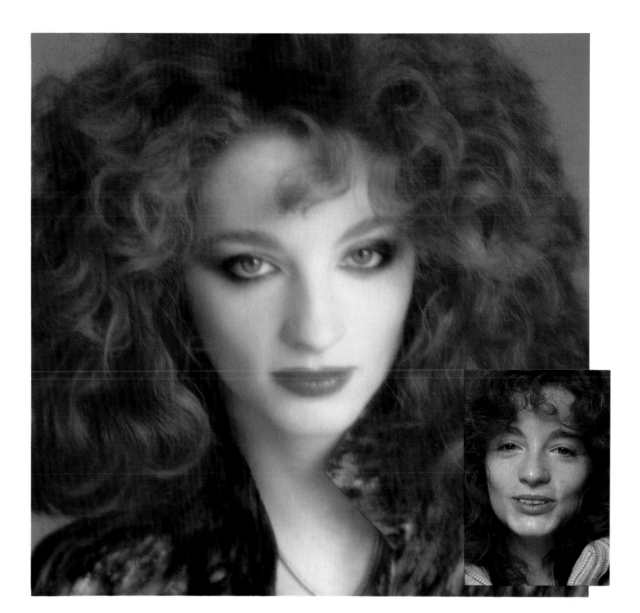

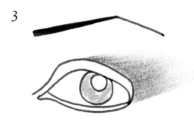

3. A *brown pencil* should then be applied quite heavily in the outer part of the eye sockets, and blended outward.

3

4. Next, apply a small line of *black kohl* in the inner upper corners of the eyes (near the nose) at the base of the lashes, and lightly under the eyes at the base of the bottom lashes. Then apply the kohl heavily in the outer upper corners and blend outward into the brown.

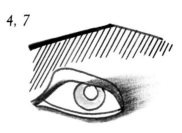

4, 7

5. Line the lips with a *bright red lip pencil*, enlarging the upper lip slightly.

6. Dust the entire face, including the eyelids, with a *transparent powder* in order to fix the penciling and keep it from creasing.

7. A *white highlighting powder* is then blended under the eyebrow over the eyebrow bone.

35

8. Blend a *pale mustard powder eye shadow* over the center of the mobile part of the eyelid, and in toward the nose.

9. Apply *black mascara* to both top and bottom lashes.

10. Line inside the rim of the lower lashes with a *black kohl pencil.*

11. Blend a *light tawny blusher* on the undersides of the cheekbones.

12. A *bright orange-red lipstick* is then applied to the lips.

8, 10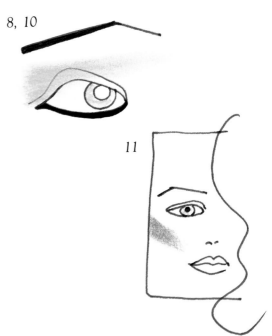

11

katy

To *modify*: The ruddy skin tone
To *accentuate*: The regal bearing
The sparkling blue eyes

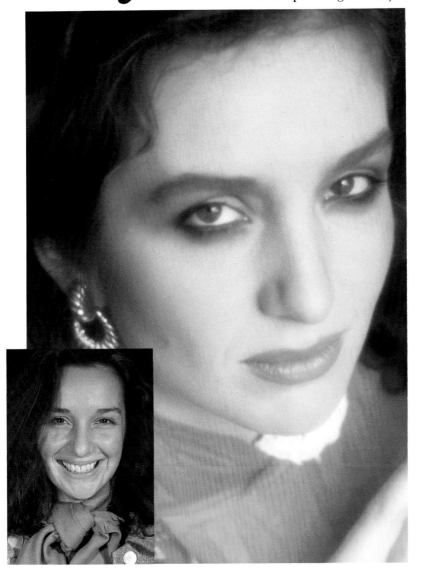

2, 7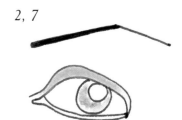

3, 6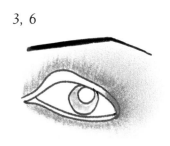

5, 9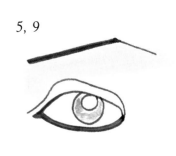

1. Apply a *beige foundation* to the entire face, including the eyelids.

2. Using a *pale turquoise pencil or cream eye shadow*, color the mobile part of the eyelid. Often, powder shadow alone is not enough when a clear color is needed. If a pencil of the same color is used first, this intensifies the shade.

3. Color the eyebrow bone with a *reddish-brown pencil*. Blend it down to the turquoise, around the turquoise at the outer corner, then under the eye at the base of the bottom lashes. Reddish-brown complements blue, and therefore reinforces the color of the eyes.

4. Powder the skin with a *transparent powder*. For a paler effect, use a white powder.

5. A *pale peach highlighter* should then be applied just under the eyebrows, on the eyebrow bone.

6. A *reddish-brown matte powder eye shadow* can then be applied sparingly over the red-brown pencil and blended into the highlighter.

7. Apply a *pale turquoise matte powder eye shadow* on top of the area already shaded in Step 2. This will intensify the color.

10

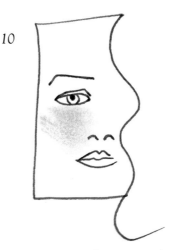

8. *Brown mascara* then is applied to top and bottom lashes.

9. Line inside the lower rim of the eyes with a *brown kohl pencil*.

10. For a softer, more romantic effect, a *light matte pink blusher* should be applied on top of the cheekbone, under the center of the eye. Avoid frosted shades.

11. A *pale lilac face powder* was used to lighten the skin even more. This is especially beautiful in the evening. In daytime, the effect is too chalky. Lilac powder is best used over another powder for a more transparent effect.

12. Draw in the lips with a *muted pink pencil*, enlarging the upper lip slightly. Follow the natural line but stay just outside it.

13. Apply a *pale pink lipstick*.

katy (2)

8

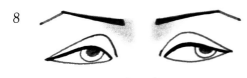

To modify: The rather large nose
The small upper lip
To accentuate: The cheekbones
The elegant, sophisticated look

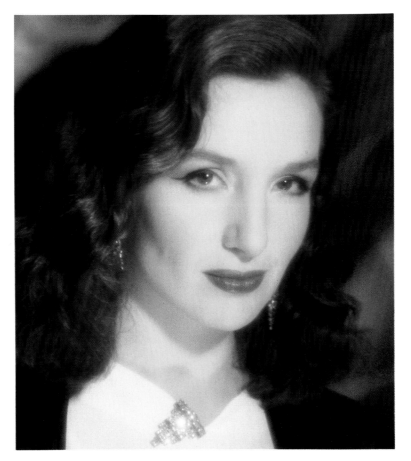

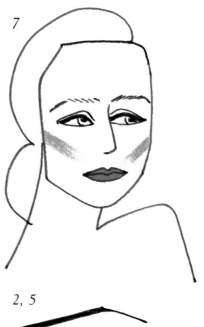

7

2, 5

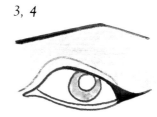

3, 4

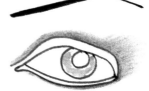

1. Apply the same *foundation* used in the previous makeover.

2. With a *dark gray pencil or powder eye shadow,* darken the eye socket, lengthening the eye slightly by blending the color outward at the outer corner.

3. Apply a *pale frosted gray powder eye shadow* to the entire eyelid.

4. *Black eyeliner* then is applied as close as possible to the base of the top lashes, widened toward the outer corner, and drawn slightly out and upward, as shown in the sketch.

5. Slightly darken the base of the bottom lashes with a *black pencil.*

6. Apply a little *white powder* to the cheekbone to highlight this area.

7. Shade the undersides of the cheekbones with a *gray-brown powder blusher.*

8. Use this same blusher to darken the eyebrow bone at the beginning of the eyebrows, the end of the nose, and the sides of the nose from halfway down, as shown. The bridge of the nose is narrow and could be lightened.

9. Use a *dark red matte lipstick,* slightly enlarging the upper lip again.

Even in Leo-governed ancient Rome, the dark-haired Roman women favored golden hair. Before a bleaching method was invented, they fashioned blond wigs

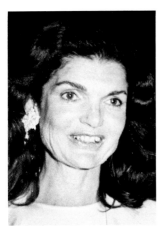

JACQUELINE ONASSIS

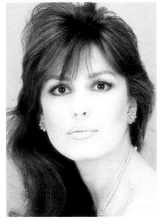

MARIA LINDBERG

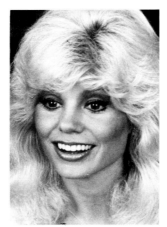

LONI ANDERSON

from the hair of Teutonic barbarian prisoners. Both men and women used cosmetics; Nero is but one notable example of a man who applied them liberally. He used ceruse (a white lead-based cosmetic) and chalk to whiten his face, Egyptian kohl to blacken his eyes and lashes, and red fucus, a paint derived from lichen, to brighten his cheeks and lips. The simply dressed, fashionable tall blond Roman woman of the epoch also had bright red cheeks, shaded her eyes with kohl or saffron, penciled her brows, and used cutout patches as beauty marks on her face and neck.

Jacqueline Onassis, with her sculpted cheekbones and wide-set eyes, is a perfect example of the strong, exotic Leo beauty. Her regal carriage was evident well before she entered the White House as First Lady. She leaves her skin very natural-looking, uses lots of mascara and a pale shade on her eyelids to bring them out a little, and she never varies from her pale, shiny lipstick. Her makeup has hardly changed over time; it suits her strong face—a face full of character—extremely well.

The enormous difference in their appearances—makeup, hair color, and style—masks the similarities between Ms. Onassis and Loni Anderson. Both have the Leonine nose—straight and well proportioned—the short, wide face and expressive eyes, as well as the radiant smile so appropriate to a sign ruled by the sun.

Ms. Anderson enlarges her already big hazel eyes with a short white line in the outer corner and a light brown shadow blended into the crease of the eye socket and at the outer corner of the eye. White highlighter just beneath the eyebrows opens up this part of the face even more. The inside lower rim of the eyes and the base of the upper lashes are usually lined with a pearly blue-turquoise, and black eyeliner is applied just at the base of the top lashes. This is followed by lots of black mascara. Her typically Leonine mouth— with the narrower upper lip—is always lined with a pencil and is very glossy, although never heavily colored. Still, the strong bright red matte lipstick so becoming to the Leo woman, along with dark smoky-gray and black eye makeup, would look equally stunning on her.

There is always a strong empathy between the two fire signs Sagittarius and Leo, so it is natural that Sagittarian designer Ronaldus Shamask chose renowned model Iman to describe his favorite type of beauty—elegant and exotic. Iman feels that the most important thing for her is eye makeup. At one time she used lots of purples and pinks, and she enjoys earth tones, but her favorite is black around the eyes and inside the lower rim, to enlarge them. She can go without blusher since her cheekbones are prominent and beautifully shaped; she feels that blusher under her cheekbones makes her face much too

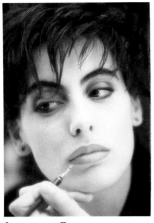 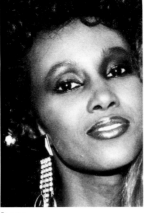

INES DE LA FRESSANGE   IMAN

hollow. Iman has found that only theatrical makeup has sufficient color for black skin. Most makeup bases are generally too yellow or red for her, so she mixes two foundations containing these tints and then dusts her face with powder, which is essential, since these foundations are quite oily. She lightly touches up her face with a tissue after applying the foundation and before dusting on the powder and, since theatrical powders are quite heavy, she applies it with a brush instead of a puff for a light effect. In the evenings, she often wears no base and just a touch of colored powder. Because of a slight discoloration, her lower lip is lighter than the upper lip, and lip gloss does not give her enough coverage. Iman has discovered that applying lipstick first, then outlining her lips with the dryer pencil, works best for her. Raw coconut oil is her favorite summer beauty product. She uses it at the beach for tanning, and then in the evening in her hair and on her face for a fabulous glow that enhances her tan even more.

Many people consider Iman the ideal African princess. With her small but wide face and fantastic bone structure, she is every bit as regal-looking as the Lioness. The same could be said of Jacqueline Onassis, who is certainly considered something of an American aristocrat.

Ines de la Fressange, like Iman, is at the top of the modeling profession because of her regal bearing and innate elegance. She is from an aristocratic French family (her grandmother is a marquise); thus, her strong Leonine character and regality have been intensified by her upbringing. Her appearance is typical of her sign: she has large round eyes, around which she uses black, grays, and browns, and likes delicately applied bright red lipstick to accentuate her brunette coloring. Her resemblance to Coco Chanel (Leo) has been noted on many occasions: she has recently become the model used exclusively to promote the Chanel couture image.

The stunning Swedish actress Maria Lindberg has the large round eyes, the mouth, and the facial structure of Leo. She does not wear makeup every day; her mood determines her look and she may feel like being glamorous even when she is doing housework. Her makeup, more intense a few years ago, is much subtler now (on the advice of her friends). She still enjoys it immensely—enlarging her eyes and making them more "dangerous"-looking with lots of black inside the lower rim. She likes to wear iridescent fuchsia eye shadow in the inner corner of her eyes, then adds a touch of that same shadow to her lips after applying lipstick. Maria does not like makeup that is perfectly applied. She wants it to look sensual and alive, so she usually applies it a couple of hours before going out and lets it sink into her skin a bit. As most people should, she varies her makeup with the seasons. During the summer she wears no foundation—only powder and blusher—on her freckled face. In winter she wears a medium-colored lightweight base to add some warmth to her skin. Her favorite lipsticks are light-colored ones—those nearest her lip color. On her cheekbones she prefers a light brown blusher.

v i r g o

august 22 – september 22

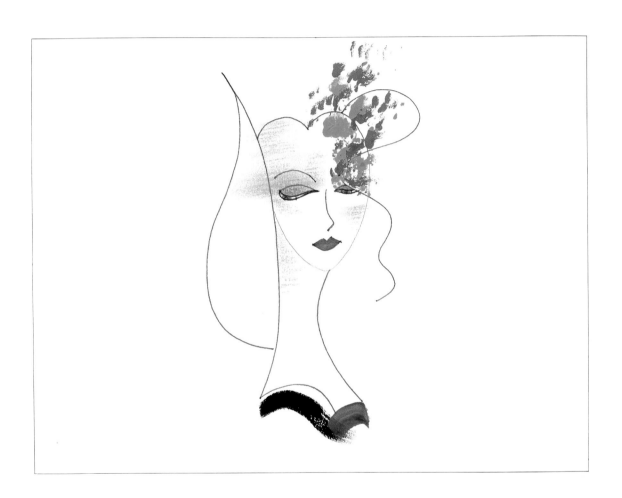

It is difficult to believe that the extremely attractive dreamer with the soft oval face and delicate cameo features could be born under the same sign as a woman with bold, piercing eyes and sharp features. The former is the most common type of Virgo, although a mixture of the two can be found. The latter type has larger eyes and a mouth which is always well defined and quite beautiful. Her features are similar to those of Pisces, her polar opposite, but are distinguished by the flatter planes of the face and the sharper-eyed, less dreamy expression. Although not as harmonious, Virgo's features are still extremely attractive, with an intriguing beauty—the kind that "grows on you."

The lovely, typically high forehead is often accentuated by a widow's peak, and the serene, slightly protruding, and heavy-lidded eyes are framed by high, delicate eyebrows. Depth should be given to the eyes by applying dark, preferably earthy, shades next to the lashes. Even those rare Virgos with deep-set eyes will find that this technique will enlarge them. Balance is the key word in all Virgo makeup, to enhance the purity and tranquillity of expression. Blues, pinks, and other bright colors on her eyes give her a harsh, painted look unless they are used sparingly and combined with the colors more flattering to her sign: rust, dark green, all shades of brown from beige to chocolate, and, for the dark-haired Virgo, black. Although it is good for her clothing, gray should be avoided as it tends to harden the Virgo woman's face.

To further accentuate harmony and softness, blusher should be kept to a minimum on the cheekbones, and a little used around the face and under the chin for a luminous effect. Light russet shades, apricot, and peach are all suitably discreet for Virgo. Her skin tone is usually very even. Some pale foundation under the eyes will highlight this area and deemphasize the slightly protruding eyelids. This plus a light dusting of transparent powder is all she will need to enhance her skin, if she has been getting enough fresh country air (her complexion's most important revitalizer).

In her youth, Virgo tends to neglect her skin, which is astonishing for such a meticulous person. This is probably because she has little or no complexion trouble and therefore assumes, incorrectly, that it is unnecessary. Although Virgos generally stay youthful-looking until late in life, the permanently anxious look, another Virgo trait, can cause frown lines on the forehead at quite a young age. A good skin-care program (the Virgo woman is usually satisfied with moderately priced, clinical-seeming products) and lessons in relaxing

facial muscles can prevent or alleviate this problem.

If foundation is applied to the entire face, a tinted moisturizer or, at most, a fine-textured foundation is best. Anything heavier will be too obvious and will coarsen this delicate face.

For both types of Virgos, the lips can be slightly enlarged. At the very least, care should be taken to extend the color right to the edge of the lips. This will lessen the doll-like effect makeup can have on the softer-faced Virgo. For the sharper-featured woman, it will add sensuality to her looks, unless she has the large, well-defined mouth, in which case this will not be necessary. A great variety of lipstick shades are available to both Virgos: russets, ambers, salmon pink, oranges, and even reds. The Virgo with the larger mouth could be even more adventurous, adding browns, mustard shades, and bluish-pinks to the above shades as well as a clear gloss, which, on the younger Virgo, creates a very interesting contrast with strongly colored eyes.

When Virgo's stone, the Mercury-governed aquamarine, is worn, the softer salmon pink and russet shades would be best. Topaz, another stone associated with Virgo, is most becoming with oranges or clear reds. It is interesting to note that sardonyx, the stone used in cameo jewelry, is also ruled by this sign. It is almost as if the first type of Virgo mentioned in this chapter—she with the delicate, dreamy expression—had been etched in the very stone governed by her ruling sign.

Note: Although the model here is blond, I have found that Virgos are more frequently brunette. These makeovers are appropriate for darker-haired women as well.

They should, however, use black instead of brown when lining the base of the lashes and inside the lower rim of the eye.

tracy

To modify: The slightly protruding eyes

To accentuate: The delicate cameo features

The fine, porcelain-like quality of the skin

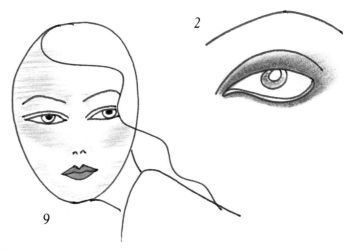

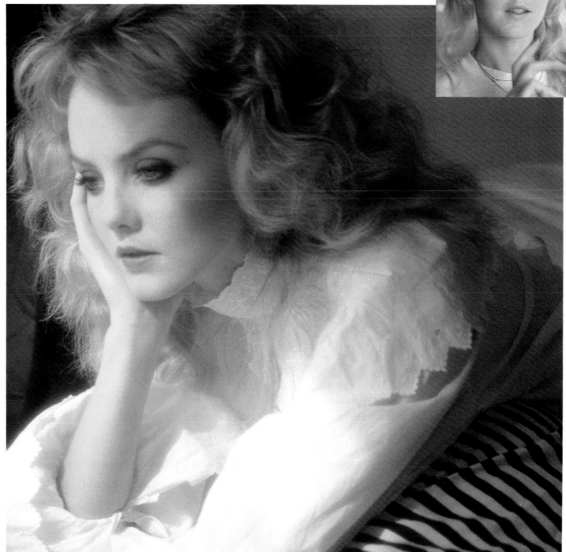

1. Apply a *very pale transparent foundation*. In this case, because of the perfect complexion, I applied only a little light foundation under the eyes and down the center of the face to highlight these areas.

2. With a *dark brown pencil*, outline the entire eye, keeping as close as possible to the eyelashes, and applying less under the eye than above. Blend slightly outward.

43

Unlik

more

much

usuall

posed

disapp

deep

color

with a

makeu

memb

a.

b.

c.

d.

1. A

v

l

e

r

2. A

e

l

c

3. (

t

i

c

a

4.

5.

8. Blend a *deep russet powder eye shadow* from the nose over the black and barely overlapping the brown. Do not cover the black shading next to the lashes or in the outer corner.

9. Apply *black mascara* to upper and lower lashes.

10. To frame the eyes well, emphasize the eyebrows with a *dark brown pencil*.

11. A *black kohl pencil* can be applied inside the rim of the lower lashes and a fine line of *black eyeliner* to the base of the upper lashes, to give more depth to the eye.

12. Blend a *deep bluish-red powder blusher* under the cheekbone onto the cheek.

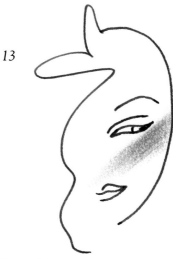

13

13. Next, blend a *deep orange-rust powder blusher* from the cheekbone into the center of the cheek.

14. Apply a *rust lipstick*. It must be much deeper and brighter than shades recommended for lighter-skinned women.

mariama (2)

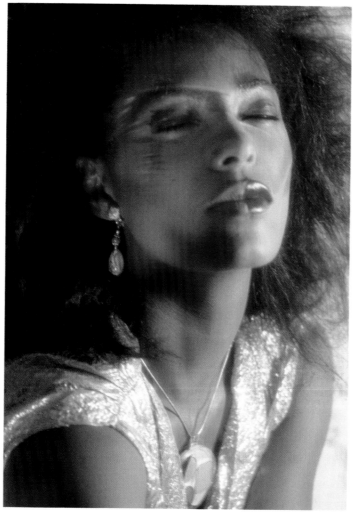

To accentuate:
The crazy side of Virgo's nature

The same base and powder used in the previous makeover are used here. Then, bright, theatrical greasepaint is used on the eyes, cheeks, and lips. Regular eye shadows are not strong enough to appear so bright on the skin. Apply these colors before powdering the face. Face powder will then fix the colors, making them longer-lasting and unsmudgeable, if you prefer this to the intense shine of the greasepaint. Fine white lines, applied with a sharp pencil, will accentuate the bright colors if placed right next to them.

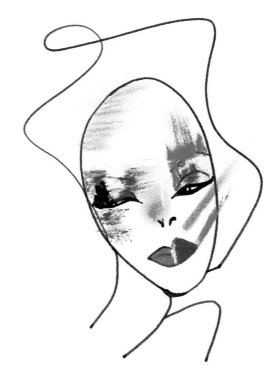

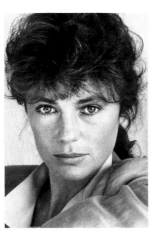

JACQUELINE BISSET

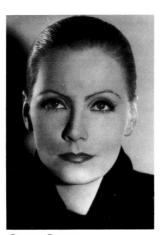

GRETA GARBO

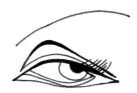

As far back as the ancient civilization of Mesopotamia, women were wearing makeup. For these women, their ruling sign, Virgo, signified purity: the purity of perfection. Natural chemists, they used macerated aromatic leaves and herbs mixed with palm and olive oils to create balms for their waxed bodies and oils to massage into their faces. They darkened their eyebrows with organic pigments, then joined them over the nose with charcoal. Mesopotamian women surrounded their eyes with a halo of blue-black antimony; a line of white lead accentuated the inner rim of their eyes. Centuries later, in Istanbul, the capital of Virgo-influenced Turkey, the eyebrows were also joined over the nose with charcoal. The eyes were lightly shaded with brown and the lips colored with a carmine tint, balancing all the features.

Greta Garbo also emphasized her finely chiseled features in a balanced way. She was the first star to tweeze her eyebrows radically and lift her eyelids and lashes to a maximum. Her look can be duplicated by whitening the entire eyelid, then darkening the eye socket with dark red, dark brown, or black. Start at the inner corner,

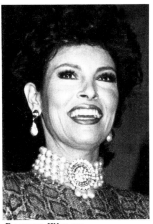
RAQUEL WELCH

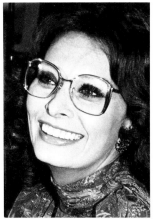
SOPHIA LOREN

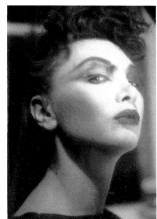
TONI BASIL

take the line quite high up over the eye socket, then descend again to almost touch the outside corner (see sketch). This line is best applied with the eye relaxed and looking straight ahead. White pencil should then be used inside the lower rim of the eye, continuing slightly outward, then inward under the tear duct. Next, use black eyeliner, beginning at the start of the white in the inner corner. Take it over the upper lashes and taper off into the white at the outer corner. A fine black line should also be drawn under the eye, joining the two outer points of the top eyeliner. Apply black mascara to upper and lower lashes. A few false eyelashes applied to the outer edge of the top lashes will complete this sultry look. The normally small Virgo mouth can be enlarged à la Garbo by darkening inside the corners of the mouth, then continuing this shading slightly, and delicately, outward. The upper lip is then outlined from the two outer points to give the mouth a slightly upturned effect. (Actually, in profile, the corners of Garbo's mouth dipped sharply when she assumed a sober expression. This somewhat severe look contrasted with the full-face effect, which was much softer.)

In the 1950s and 1960s, Italian beauty Sophia Loren used eye makeup much as Garbo did. She gave depth to her eyes with shading, then lengthened them with eyeliner and false eyelashes, often using that touch of white at the outer corners between, and joining, the upper and lower lines. Her eyebrows were drawn in, hair by hair, with typical Virgoan precision. Raquel Welch, with facial features similar to Ms. Loren's, has used the same precision in her own perfectly balanced makeup.

Michael Jackson also uses makeup in the discreet Virgoan manner. He lightens his skin tone slightly, which is very effective in catching the light (although I would recommend a base with a warmer undertone, as his has a tendency to look grayish). To add more depth to his eyes, the base of his bottom lashes is darkened, as are the mobile parts of his heavy-lidded Virgo eyes. He also shades the sides and tip of his nose for further dimension.

Singer Toni Basil, on the other hand, loves to experiment, and her crazy Virgo curiosity inspires her to try anything. Her large, slightly protruding eyes and beautiful bone structure make her the perfect model for the latest, most extravagant makeup look.

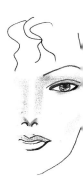

l i b r a

september 23 – october 22

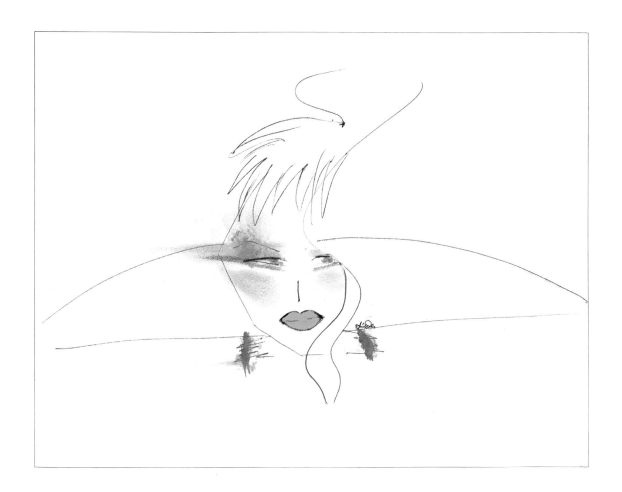

Elegance and refinement are the two outstanding qualities of Libra, who, like Taurus, is governed by Venus. In her quest for perfection, Libra effortlessly lends a physical form to the ideal of beauty in all she does. She instinctively knows how to maintain and express her beauty, and takes great care of herself. As a result, Libra appears confident and knowing, and the strong charm and agreeable expression that arise from this self-confidence make her very attractive and almost always pretty.

When Venus is strong in the charts of other signs, it softens the physical features of those signs. Conversely, the normally soft features of the Libran are easily modified by other astrological influences in her chart. As a matter of fact, her physical traits often seem to be taken completely from the more powerful, distinctive signs in her horoscope.

Colors fascinate the Libra woman, but her aesthetic sense leads her away from opulence in favor of harmony and elegance. She can adapt even the most difficult and unusual makeup to her own looks while retaining her sensuality and char-

49

acter. Because of this, there is no hard and fast rule for her makeup. She should follow her intuition. Libran-ruled colors such as soft blues and pastels are very flattering; no other sign is able to use them with such subtlety and warmth. While Taurus is an earth sign ruled by Venus, and therefore most attractive in earthier colors and paler pinks, Libra is an air sign, able to use all shades of pink to enhance her Venus-bestowed charms. From a soft pink when she is feeling soft and cuddly to a sexy shocking pink to a deep, sensual pinkish burgundy for her more vampish moods, the color pink seems to have been created with Libra in mind. To emphasize her special refined beauty, Libra can balance bluish-pink lipstick with mustard and copper shades.

Many eye shapes are found among Librans. The two that I find most common are featured below. If your eyes are different, consult the technical index at the back of the book for your particular shape and insert Libra colors into those instructions.

The Libran face is often heart-shaped, slightly hexagonal, with the forehead somewhat narrower than the jaw. The prominent cheekbones form the widest part of the face. The eyebrows are gracefully arched and not usually very strong. Libra's delicate skin is a mirror of her physical and emotional health; dark circles under the eyes and a lifeless complexion appear after a depressed period or an active partying stage. These can be alleviated by occasional intensive treatments and alternating an oxygenating cream with the usual nourishing night cream. It is also important to use a deep-cleansing mask once a week to reinvigorate the complexion. Like Cancer, Libra has a tendency to sunburn easily, so extra care must be taken outdoors. Foundation will help protect the skin, and a shade slightly lighter than the skin tone, with a touch of rose in it, would be perfect for livening it up. Powder is equally important, as a matte finish is the most flattering to Librans.

The transparency of the diamond, Libra's stone, allows her the freedom to choose and intensify her makeup colors, but she has other options as well. White jade, flattering to her skin color, integrates beautifully with the refined coloring of mustard eyes and pale pink lips. When coral, the stone governed by Venus, is worn with contrasting shades of pink, it adds warmth and balance to the more bluish-pink shades. Together they reflect the harmony and elegance of the Libra beauty.

cornelia

To modify: The slightly drooping eyes
The rather thin upper lip
The dull skin tone
To accentuate: The prominent cheekbones
The sensual side of the Libran beauty

1. Apply *light beige foundation* to the entire face, including the eyelids. It should be as close in color as possible to the neck, which in this case is extremely beautiful.

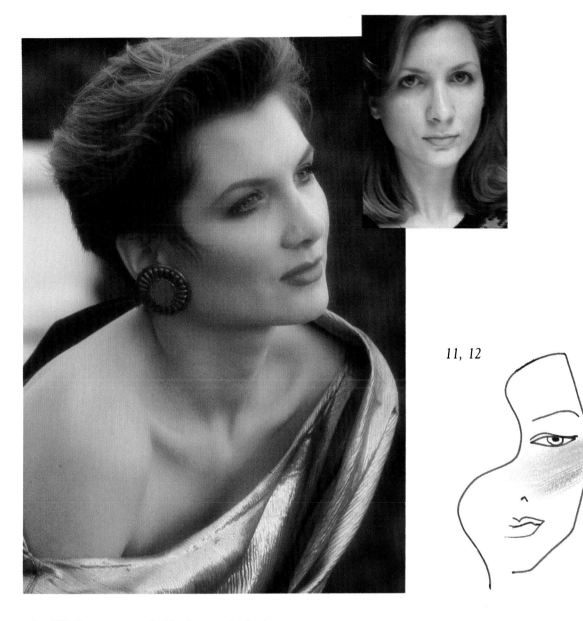

11, 12

2. With a very soft *black pencil*, darken the base of the upper and lower lashes in the outer corner of the eyes and blend outward.

2, 4, 7

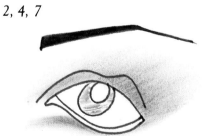

3. Take a *burgundy pencil* and apply on top of the black, blending it further out and upward. Under the eye, blend it down toward the nose. This is very important for drooping eyes, as the downward line raises the outer corner (see sketch).

3

4. Lighten the inner corner of the eye with a *white or light pink pencil*.

5. With a *dark pink pencil*, outline the lips, enlarging the upper lip slightly as shown. Blend with a lipbrush for a softer effect.

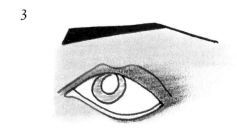

5

51

6. Powder the entire face liberally with *transparent powder*—especially the penciled part of the eye.

7. Apply a *light pink frosted eye shadow* on the lids near the nose, blending outward.

8. Beginning on the pale pink at the center of the eyelid, blend a *darker frosted pink shadow* outward, covering the penciled black and burgundy.

9. Apply *black mascara* to both top and bottom lashes.

10. Brushing and using short sharp strokes, thicken the eyebrows slightly with a *taupe pencil*. With strong eye makeup it's essential that eyebrows be well shaped and colored.

8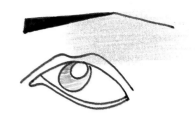

11. Apply a *light brown matte blusher* under the cheekbones, blending down.

12. Then apply *light pink blusher* on the cheekbones themselves.

13. Apply a *bright salmon-pink lipstick* (rather than bluish-pink) to warm up the overall effect.

Note: Both of the following makeovers are designed for oblique (upturned) eyes. If your eyes droop, then the color on the lids should be darker toward the outer edge and lightened in the inner corner, as in the previous makeover.

laura

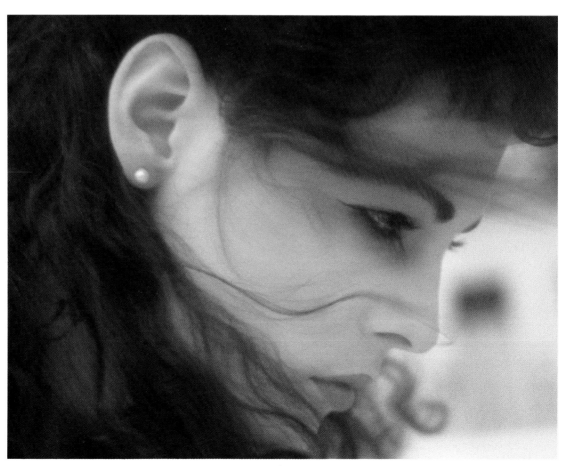

1. Apply a *very pale foundation.*

2. To make the eye seem Eastern, it is easier to begin by narrowing it with kohl—black or otherwise—inside the lower rim. In this case, a *reddish-brown kohl pencil* was used.

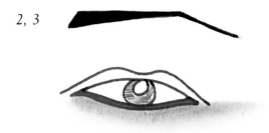

2, 3

3. Blend the same color kohl under the eye and straight out to further lengthen it.

4. Cover the entire eyelid with a *pale bluish-gray cream or powder shadow,* blending it up and outward to the eyebrows.

4

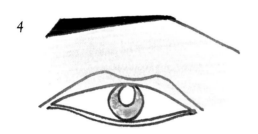

5. Powder the face and eyelids with a *pale or transparent powder.*

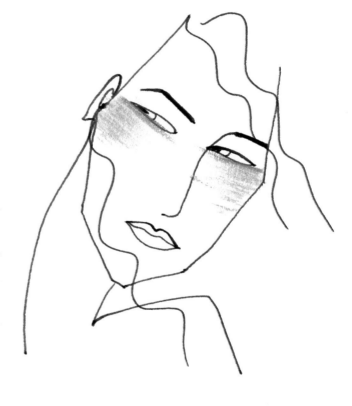

6. For a stronger makeup, another layer of blue-gray eye shadow can be added on the lid.

7. Apply a *bright orange powder blusher* high on the cheekbones, blending it in with the reddish-brown under the eyes.

8. Lengthen the eyes with a very fine line of *black liquid eyeliner.* Take care not to lift the line, but take it out straight (see sketch). If your eyes are round, you can make them narrower by lining under the eyes only. Begin just beneath the inner corner and draw it straight out. No mascara is used, as it opens the eyes too much.

8

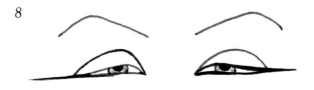

9. Outline the lips with a *red pencil.*

10. Fill in the lips with an *orange-red lipstick.*

laura (2)

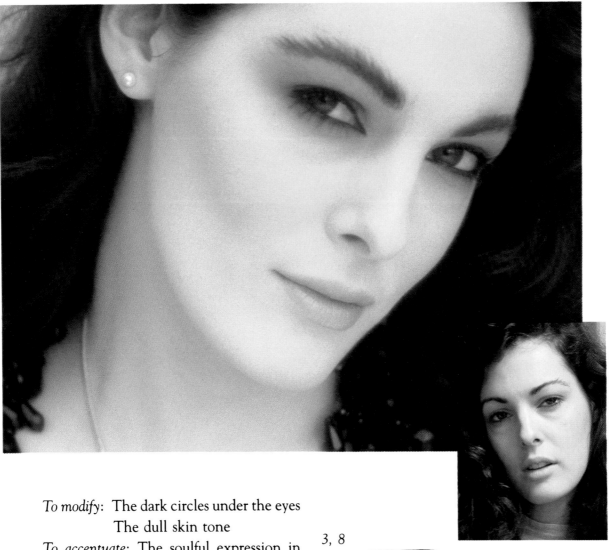

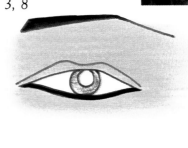

To *modify*: The dark circles under the eyes
           The dull skin tone

To *accentuate*: The soulful expression in
           the eyes
           The refined Libran beauty

3, 8

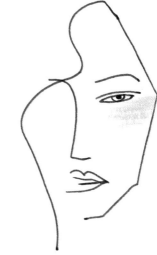

9

1. With a fine clean brush, apply some *concealer* to the dark lines under the eyes.

2. Cover the entire face, including the eyelids, with *very pale foundation*.

3. Apply *mustard powder or cream eye shadow* to the entire eyelid and under-eye area. Begin close to the lashes and blend outward and up to the eyebrows. The color will be slightly stronger at the outer corner.

4. Powder the entire face liberally with a *light-colored or transparent powder*, not

forgetting the eyelid and under the eyes.

5. Brush the face to remove excess powder.

6. If a stronger effect is desired, apply *mustard powder* on top of the already colored area.

7. Apply *black mascara* to top and bottom lashes.

8. Line inside the lower rim of the eyes with a *black kohl pencil.*

9. Blend some *light pink blusher* lightly on the top of the cheekbones.

10. Brush the eyebrows and fill them in with a finely sharpened *dark brown pencil.*

11. Apply a *pale pink tinted lip gloss*—a perfect color for these well-shaped lips.

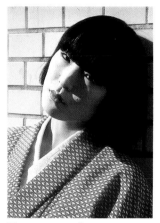

TRADITIONAL JAPANESE

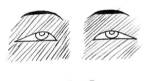

The traditional Japanese ritual of applying makeup is as beautiful and refined as the makeup itself. It is not surprising, then, to discover that Japan falls under the influence of Libra. After covering the hair with a skullcap in preparation for the wig, a special grease is massaged into the skin. The eyebrows are hidden with a concealing wax similar to the modeling wax used in Western theatrical makeup. White liquid foundation, prepared from a chalk-like stick mixed with water, is then applied with a dampened flat white brush, then blended with a wider, dry brush. Next, more white foundation is applied to the bridge of the nose. The eyebrows are drawn with a slanted brush dipped in a near-black grease, then pressed gently to blend the undersides of the lines and set the color. Another flat brush is used to apply a pastel-pink shade to the entire eyelid, a color blended down the sides of the face as well, followed by more white applied upward from the neck. White powder is then dusted on the bridge of the nose, and, more lightly, on the rest of the face. To add a touch of shading, a beige powder is used on certain parts of the face. Traditional Japanese makeup is distinguished by a dark red grease which is pressed into the inner corners of the eyes with the forefinger in a short downward stroke, then at the outer corner in a bow shape, enlongating the eye. The final step in the eye makeup is the use of black eyeliner in a very narrow line, staying above the red at the outer corner. More red is then blended into the eyebrows, and the lips are painted small and bow-shaped, with the lower lip much thicker than the upper.

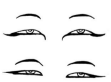

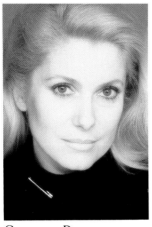

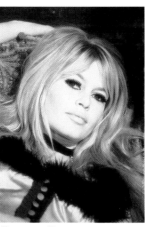

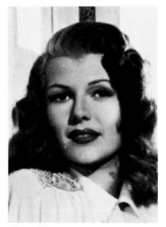

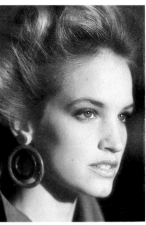

CATHERINE DENEUVE   BRIGITTE BARDOT   RITA HAYWORTH   BONNIE BERMAN

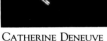

The total effect is quintessentially Libran—a harmonic and fragile elegance achieved despite the dramatic use of much makeup.

Brigitte Bardot is a typical example of the Venus-governed Libran beauty. While black eyeliner was her trademark in her youth, she developed a different, softer technique to emphasize her sensuality. She darkens her entire eyelid with dark brown, blended slightly upward to lengthen the eye. Black kohl is used inside the lower rim of the eye, followed by lots of black mascara on the upper and lower lashes. To obtain the famous Bardot pout, enlarge the outline of your lips with a light brown pencil, then apply a bit of white under the outer corners of your lips (see sketch). After applying a very pale beige matte lipstick, blend some more white into the center of the lower lip.

The wonderfully photogenic face of French actress Catherine Deneuve needs only gentle highlighting. Her delicate beauty is enhanced by a pale foundation, very close to her own skin tone. A light brown blusher under the cheekbones, with a lighter blusher just above, accentuates the shape of her face. While her eye makeup has changed with the fashions, her preference is for deep violets, purples, and brownish-plum colors as well as khaki—all of which accentuate her golden-green eyes. The base of her upper lashes is usually lined with a black pencil for further definition.

Richard Avedon (Venus-governed Taurus) and Arthur Elgort (Gemini) are two great photographers known for their appreciation of women's beauty and their ability to capture the excitement of that beauty on film. They are both especially intrigued by Libran model Bonnie Berman. Bonnie loves experimenting with makeup and instinctively knows what's best for her. Her favorite makeup is a Grace Kelly style, featuring dark shading above the eyes and well-shaped bright orange lips.

Rita Hayworth is a wonderful example of the Libran with a perfectly heart-shaped face and narrow forehead. Her wide-set eyes are flecked with changing colors of green and gold, lending a sparkling elegance to her beauty.

scorpio

october 23 – november 21

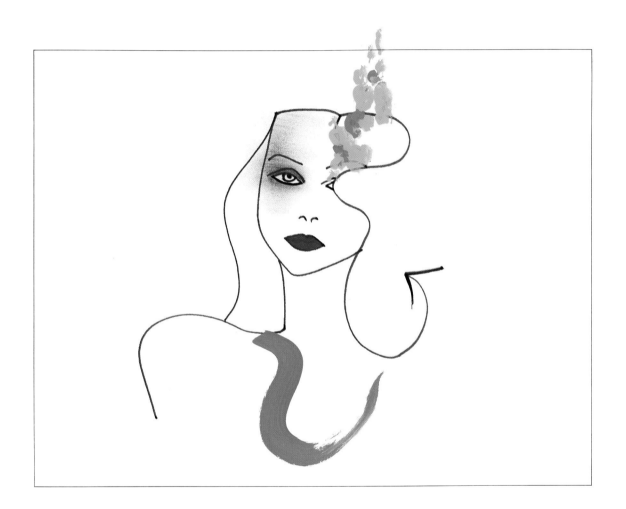

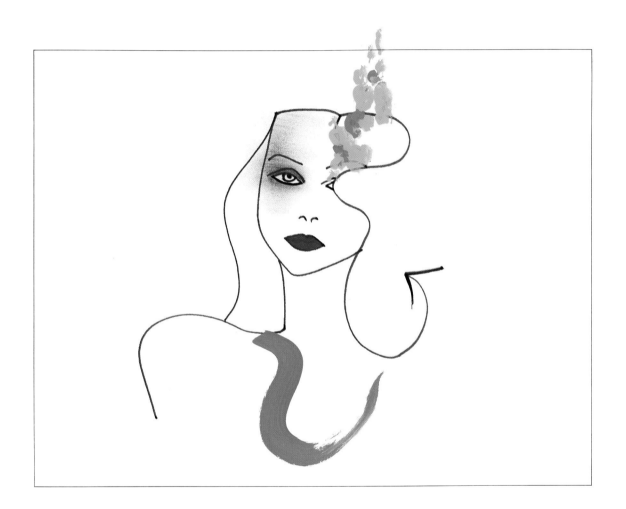 The beauty of Scorpio women is deep and mysterious, heightened by the intense magnetism of their usually round, prominent eyes. They are most often dark-haired, with dark brown, nearly black eyes. Their foreheads are generally not very high, and their jawbones are large; but with rather full cheeks and full, round lips, Scorpios have a very youthful appearance. Another fairly common Scorpio type has red hair, freckled skin, and sharper features, with a larger nose and more angular jaw. Often a mixture of these two is found. Much less common, but just as much a Scorpio, is the cool, blond, Grace Kelly type.

The Scorpio complexion, even when fair, is usually strong and not prone to many problems. If, however, Scorpio uses her inner strength and drive in a self-destructive way, her normally intelligent skin-care routine will become erratic and her hectic night life will show its effect on her complexion, especially if she has the fragile skin of the redhead, and her looks can alternate between vibrant and worn out.

Scorpios are frequently found wearing

no makeup, but because of the intensity of their appearance, they still look mesmerizing. However, they believe in anything that will strengthen their already considerable powers and enjoy makeup because it does precisely that. They wear it well, never overdoing it, as Scorpio is also a sign of self-control. Scorpios are extremely memorable individuals (although in retrospect the special ingredients of their charm cannot be precisely identified): and, while cosmetics enhance a Scorpio woman's sensuality, makeup is not the most obvious part of her appeal.

Nothing is better for her eyes than black or burgundy to emphasize their mystery, or deep, dark greens like the deep water Scorpio represents. Brighter blues and greens, on the other hand, are flattering for her lighter moods. For blushers and contouring, she should choose dark maroon or russet shades. Muted pinks also work well for her, on the cheekbones or framing the face. Her lips do not need much definition; in any case, a liner would

be too intense for her. Burgundy, pale muted pinks, or even a natural gloss would be best. Scorpio's pale skin really needs no foundation or, at the very most, a transparent one.

Bloodstones, a precious jewel ruled by Scorpio, are most flattering worn with harmonizing burgundy eye makeup, and black kohl pencil inside the lower rim of the eyes blended into the base of the lashes (see Allyson's second makeover in this section). Kohl is the most important part of Scorpio's makeup. It was invented for her, to enhance the magnetism of her already seductive eyes, and is flattering even when worn alone. Jade and topaz, also falling under the influence of Scorpio, are equally complimentary and harmonize with any of her colors. The paler, clear topaz, worn with a mixture of blues and greens, is especially original and attractive. This subtle style of makeup and jewelry accentuates the aura of intensity which makes the Scorpio woman so uniquely stunning.

patricia

To modify: The fullness of the face
The swollen eyelids

To accentuate: The penetrating Scorpio eyes
Scorpio's strong sensuality

1. Blend a little *pale foundation* over the entire face, including the eyelids.

2. With a *black pencil*, darken the base of the top and bottom lashes. Apply it a little more heavily in the top outer corner. Blend this up and outward.

3. With a *pale transparent powder*, powder the entire face, including the eyelids.

4. Apply a *matte white or pale mustard-beige eye shadow* to the eyebrow bone, just under the brows.

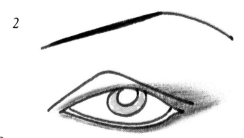

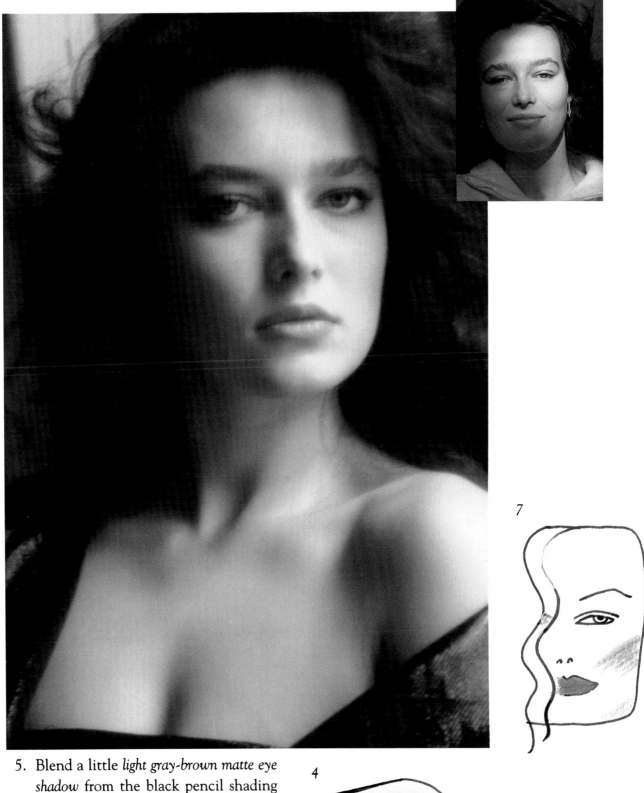

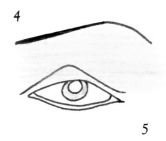

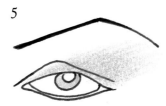

5. Blend a little *light gray-brown matte eye shadow* from the black pencil shading into the beige highlighter under the brow.

6. Apply *black mascara* to top and bottom lashes.

7. Use a little *brown matte blusher* under the cheekbone. Blend it inward toward the center of the cheeks, and down toward the corners of the mouth.

8. Use a *muted pink matte blusher* over the brown, taking it gently to the center of the cheeks.

9. Define the lips with a *pinkish-beige pencil*, then use the same color lipstick.

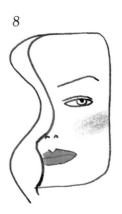

allyson

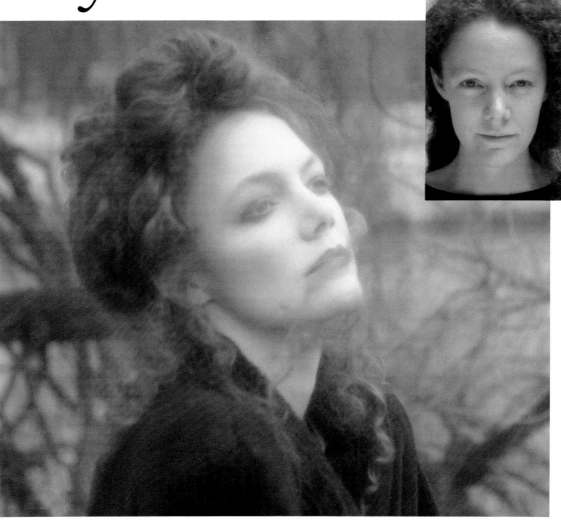

To modify: The rather angular face
To accentuate: The magnetic Scorpio eyes
The whiteness of the skin

Allyson's strong Aquarian ascendant has slightly modified her Scorpio features, especially her forehead, which is much larger than that of the average Scorpio. Here I have accentuated the mysterious quality of her sign.

1. For this extremely pale face, a little *white foundation* should be mixed with the *palest beige foundation*, then applied to the entire face, including the eyelids.

60

2. A *dark, but quite bright, blue pencil* should then be applied, as near as possible to the base of the bottom lashes, then blended down and out. Then blend up and around a little into the outer edge of the eye socket.

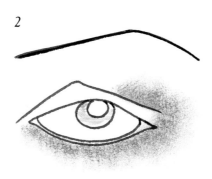

3. A *bright green cream eye shadow* should then be blended from the upper lashes over the mobile part of the lids, then up and out toward the eyebrows. A theatrical makeup will have to be used, as it is difficult to find such a bright green in commercial makeup brands.

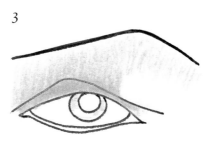

4. A *white face powder* should be dusted over the face and eyelids, taking special care on the green shading.

5. Use a *yellow powder eye shadow* under the eyebrows, to soften the finish of the green. No mascara should be used. The lack of it emphasizes, in the red-haired Scorpio, the unusual intensity of the eyes (just as kohl pencil does for the darker-haired Scorpio).

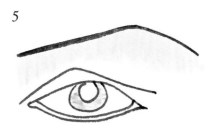

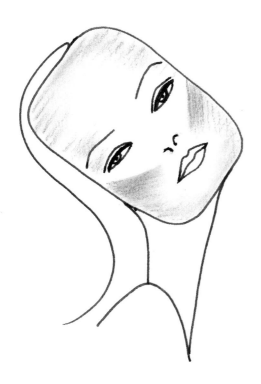

6. A *tawny blusher* should then be blended around the whole of the hairline, the jawbone, and under the cheekbones. This not only reduces the size of the face and softens the angles but also adds a little of the warmth of the hair color to the rather white face.

7. Use a *bright red lip pencil* to line the lips.

8. Apply a *bright orange lipstick* to the lips with a lipbrush.

allyson (2)

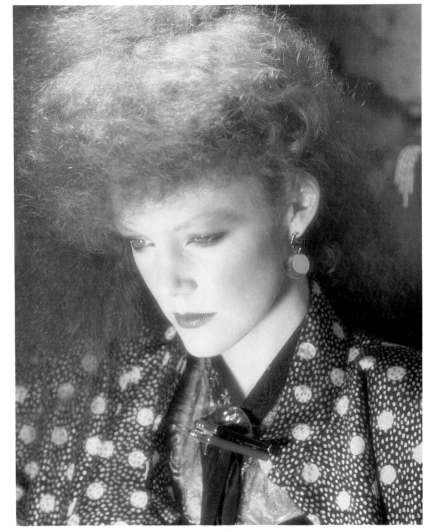

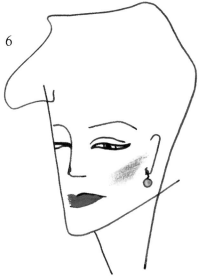

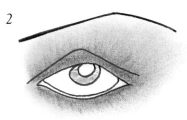

1. Apply the same base and powder as in steps 1 and 4 in the previous makeover.

2. A *deep burgundy eye shadow*—either pencil, cream, or powder—should be applied as close as possible to the bottom and top lashes. Blend up to the eyebrows, outward a little, and down under the bottom lashes. Keep the color as dark as possible next to the lashes.

3. A *pale frosted gray-pink eye shadow* should then be applied under the eyebrows near the nose. Blend well.

4. Apply *black mascara* to top and bottom lashes.

5. Line inside the lower rim of the eyes

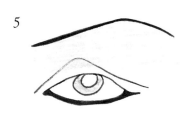

with a *black kohl pencil.*

6. A *medium shade of muted pink powder blusher* should be blended low on the cheekbone and inward toward the center of the cheek. Take care not to lengthen the face by taking the color too far down.

7. Use a *light burgundy lipstick* to finish the makeup, after first lining the lips with a *burgundy pencil.*

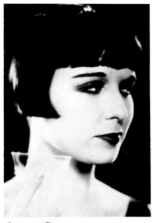

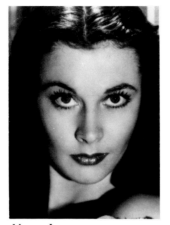

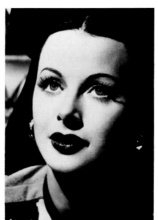

LOUISE BROOKS   VIVIEN LEIGH   HEDY LAMARR

Although a passionate sign, Scorpio is also extremely secretive—and what better way to strengthen one's mysterious aura than to wear a veil? The yashmak is still worn in Scorpio-ruled Arab countries, not only reinforcing the seclusion and mystery of Arab women but also allowing them to use to the fullest their strongest assets: piercing, hypnotizing eyes. Kohl is used almost universally, and the lips are colored with a dark ruby red—a makeup that has changed little with time.

The non-veiled, paler-skinned Berber women of Morocco also wear kohl, often using it to lengthen their eyes in unusual ways. Frequently the forehead, chin, and occasionally the tip of the nose are tattooed with blue-gray markings of varying significance. The lips are rarely colored, but the cheeks are sometimes roughened or decorated with red and black markings.

Screen star Louise Brooks was the New Woman of the twenties—confident in her image and unaffected by the opinions of others. Her eyes, surrounded by black makeup, and her sleek black hair, bobbed and brilliant as lacquer, were set off by the incredibly pure whiteness of her skin. The box-office favorite of the forties was sultry Veronica Lake, obviously a Scorpio be-

cause of her "veil"—the peekaboo hairstyle for which she was so famous.

Alfred Hitchcock once described Grace Kelly's special appeal as "sexual elegance." The cool refinement of her flawless complexion, superb bone structure, and perfect white teeth could not hide completely the deeper spirit of the secretive, magnetic Scorpio.

Television star Linda Evans falls into the same Scorpio category as Grace Kelly. She is well aware that minimal makeup is all she needs to enhance her beauty, and wears a combination of blacks, browns, and grays on her eyes to obtain an effect similar to Patricia's makeup, as described earlier in this chapter. Ms. Evans' healthy, tanned skin and glossy lips give her a different but equally attractive overall look. Designer Anne Marie Beretta (Libra) finds that her ideal beauty is a strong, elegant woman whose exterior is in harmony with her inner nature. She names Katharine Hepburn as a perfect example. Ms. Hepburn is the quintessential red-haired Scorpio with a strong jaw, angular features, and penetrating, smoky blue-green eyes. She never wears makeup, but remains striking to this day without it.

The entire history of the silver screen,

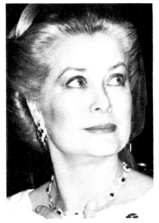
GRACE KELLY

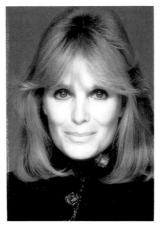
LINDA EVANS

in fact, would be far less rich and glamorous without the Scorpio mystique. Vivien Leigh created a sensation by virtue of her sheer physical beauty. She was tiny and fragile, with the pale complexion perfect for the Southern beauties she portrayed, and her enormous cat's eyes were perfect for her roles as a tempestuous seductress. Considered by her contemporaries to be one of the greatest beauties of her time, Ms. Leigh, clad in the soft, deep garnet of the mesmerizing Scorpio, played the romantic sirens of fact and fiction as no other actress could.

sagittarius

november 22 – december 21

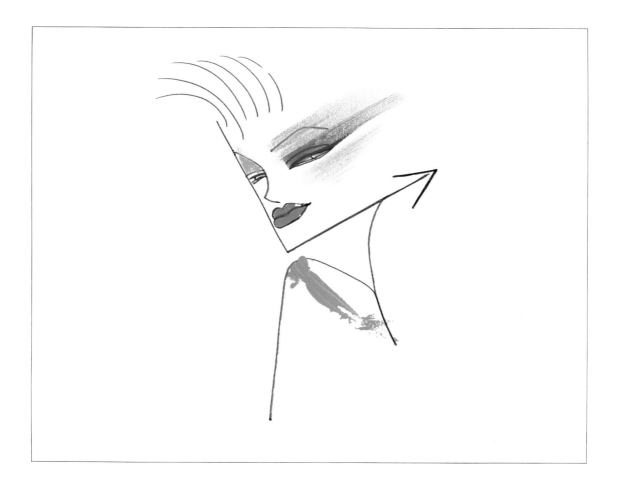

Sagittarius is the bright, breezy, joyful beauty of the zodiac. She has an engaging smile and is naturally healthy-looking, if she has learned to control her love of food and drink. Even if she is blond or auburn-haired, as most Sagittarians are, she'll often have a slightly tanned complexion. Her best beauty treatment is the fresh air in which she seems to have been bred, and a good moisturizer, since her skin will probably be prone to dryness.

A comparatively large skull and wide face and forehead are typical Sagittarian traits and combine to give her an alert, candid look. She has perfect almond-shaped eyes which are slightly upturned; well-defined, gently arched brows; and a small nose. Although her mouth is usually narrow, it too is beautifully shaped, with a slight upward lift in the corners, and her exceptional smile is made all the more attractive by her perfect white teeth. Even when not openly smiling, Sagittarius has a sparkling, mischievous look about the eyes and mouth.

Sagittarius enjoys following the latest trends in makeup. She is an impulsive and extravagant buyer and often purchases products without taking the time to make sure they are right for her. As a result, she will often make mistakes. To avoid them, her motto should be "the simpler the better," for her natural beauty and the charm of her fine features can be drowned by the wrong colors or too heavy a hand. No more than two eye shadows are usually necessary on the eyelids, blended to avoid harsh contrasts, and taken softly up and outward, following the oblique lines of the eye. Muted violets, greens, and browns—preferably matte, but at most slightly iridescent—are most flattering to her. Violet, especially, will enhance her more sophisticated side, as will eyeliner, to emphasize the fantastic shape of her eyes. For a less formal look, though, darkening only the base of the bottom lashes with brown pencil is wonderfully effective.

Heavy, dark, or harsh bright colors should be avoided, with the exception of orange, which is as lovely on her eyes as it is on her lips. Many Sagittarians use pink eye shadow along with bright bluish-pink on their lips and cheeks. This is a classic case of "overkill." Sagittarius simply does not need all that color—it sharpens her features and drowns her most entrancing quality—her sunny warmth.

To keep that warmth in her complexion, then, Sagittarius should use a russet or peachy shade of blusher, or a golden brown, even when using violet eye shadow. And, as in the eye makeup, lightness of hand should be the rule. Healthy golden foundation colors are best, unless the skin is very pale. If the complexion has a lightly tanned look, a tinted moisturizer may be all she needs. This, along with mascara, a cream blusher on the cheekbones, and a lip gloss are perfect for the sporty Sagittarius who wants only to enhance her natural good looks. A light dusting of face powder to tone down shininess, and lipstick instead of gloss, transform this into city makeup. Sagittarians have a wide choice of lipstick shades. Along with beiges and russets, they look good in bright pinks, violets, oranges, and reds.

The extroverted beauty of Sagittarius enables her to wear all red and green stones well. Her most flattering stone is amethyst, which is governed by her ruling planet, Jupiter, and which harmonizes beautifully with any of the above-mentioned makeup colors. Turquoise is another attractive option, for a more casual look. The coolness of the stone against her warm complexion perfectly emphasizes the fresh vitality of the Sagittarian beauty and disposition.

barbara

Note: Even though this face is rather wide, it is much too smiling and expressive to call for resculpturing.

To accentuate: The glowing warmth of the Sagittarian personality

1. A *natural beige foundation* should be used sparingly on the entire face.

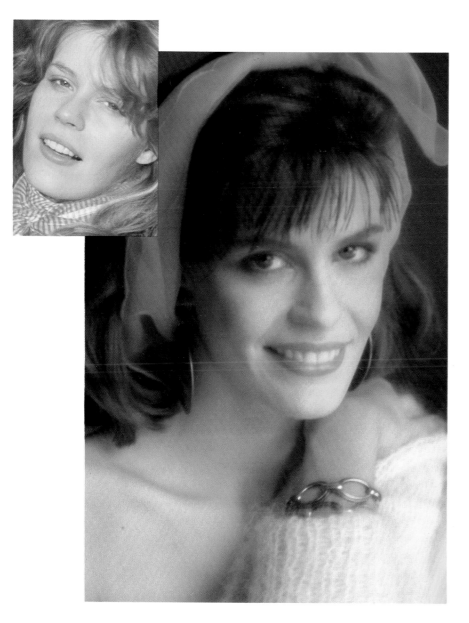

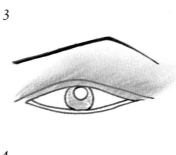

7

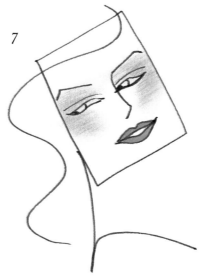

2. Lightly dust the face with a *transparent powder*.

3. An *orange powder or cream eye shadow* should be blended lightly from the base of the eyelashes up and outward to the eyebrows.

4. Next, blend a *dark reddish-brown powder eye shadow* from the base of the lashes to the outer upper corners of the eyes.

5. Apply *brown mascara* to both top and bottom lashes.

6. Brush the eyebrows slightly upward.

7. Apply *orange powder or cream blusher* to the cheekbones.

3

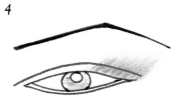

4

8. Apply an *orange lipstick*, similar to the orange shade used on the eyes.

67

lari

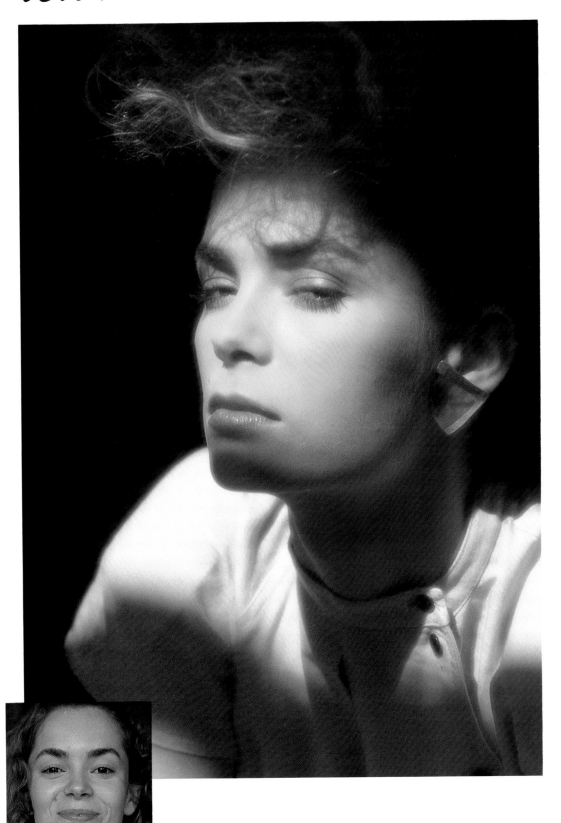

To modify: The slightly angular face
The troubled complexion
To accentuate: The refreshing, modern
Sagittarian personality

1. Apply a *creamy golden foundation* to the face and neck. The neck should never be left darker than the face.

2. Apply to each blemish, with a small brush, a *light shade of concealer* (or a light shade of Clinique Continuous Coverage). Blend well, and on top of this apply more foundation to help blend further. If there are many blemishes, a foundation with heavier coverage should be used.

3

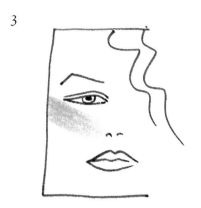

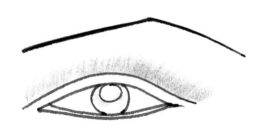

6

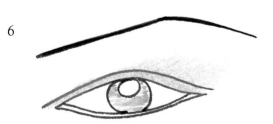

7, 8

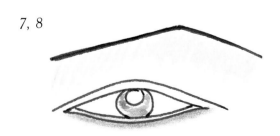

3. Blend a *creamy amber-colored blusher* on the cheekbones. If they are broken out, you may have to touch up the blemishes again with a brush before proceeding.

4. Apply a *medium brown eye shadow* in the crease of the eye and blend outward.

5. Before applying powder, make sure the blemishes do not appear darker than the rest of the face. It's better for them to appear slightly lighter, if not exactly the same color. Then dust the entire face and eyelids with a *transparent powder*, pressing it gently into the foundation so that the coverage is not disturbed. Remove excess powder with a very soft brush.

6. Blend a *slightly iridescent muted violet eye shadow* over the eyelid outward into the brown shading.

7. Apply a touch of *cream-colored powder eye shadow* to the eyebrow bone.

8. Slightly darken the base of the bottom lashes with a *brown pencil*.

9. Apply *brown mascara* to top and bottom lashes.

10. Use *transparent lip gloss* on the lips.

lari (2)

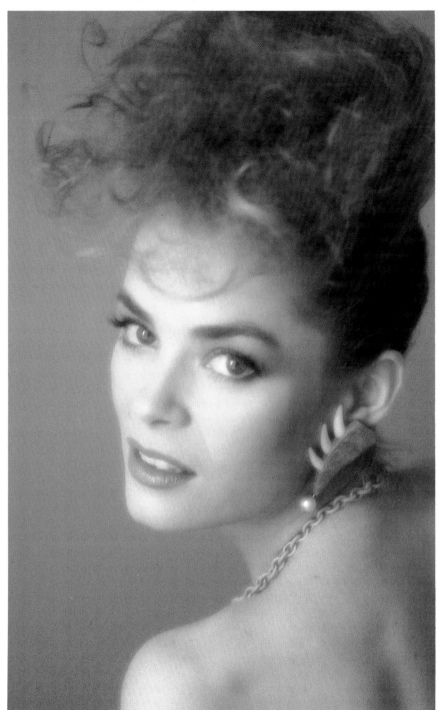

Perform Steps 1 through 4 as in previous makeover.

5. Blend a *bronze powder eye shadow* over the eyebrow bone just under the brow.

6. Apply a *muted green powder eye shadow* from the lashes over the lid and onto the bronze powder.

5

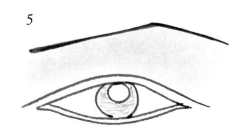

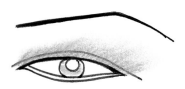

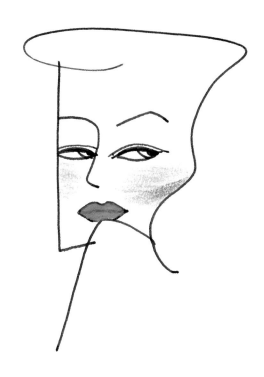

7. Finely line the base of the upper lashes with *dark brown liquid eyeliner*.

8. In the outside upper corner of the eyes, apply three or four small clusters of *false eyelashes* to the base of the real lashes, making them slightly longer toward the outside. This will exaggerate the naturally oblique shape of the eyes.

9. Enlarge the upper lip slightly with *dark pink lip pencil*, making it rounder and more sensual. Blend the pencil line with a brush.

10. Apply a *bright pink lipstick* with a lip-brush for better definition.

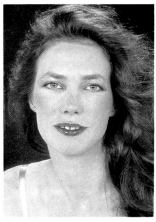

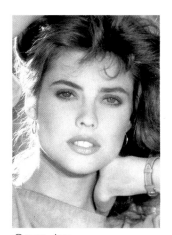

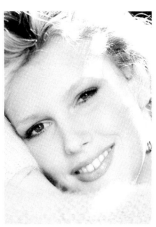

JANE BIRKIN   CAROL ALT   CARRIE NYGREN

The gregarious, wonderfully healthy-looking women of Australia epitomize the nature of Sagittarius, their ruling sign. Australia, the land of open spaces and wide frontiers, is also a land of open faces and active, outdoorsy inhabitants. Still, anyone who has visited Australia's major cities knows that the Australians are also extremely fashionable—the recent "Australian invasion" in film and music is proof of that. The women have a great love for makeup and are very up-to-date in their use of cosmetics, at times (in true Sagittarian style) using a bit too much of a good thing.

Actress and singer Jane Birkin's long, rectangular face, almond eyes, and mobile features are typical of her sign, although her smooth complexion is paler than that of the average Sagittarian. She wears very

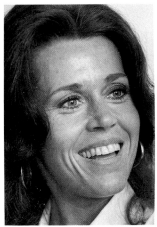
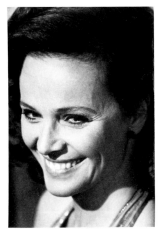

JANE FONDA   LAURA ANTONELLI

little makeup, but her beauty—casual and naturally sensuous—is more eye-catching because of it.

Model Carrie Nygren has a strong Gemini rising, which gives her a lovely widow's peak and a more pointed chin than most Sagittarians. When doing her own makeup, Carrie opens up her narrow almond-shaped eyes by applying a soft russet shade of blusher above the crease line of the eye socket, and a harder color—usually fuchsia or dark gray—in the outer corners of the eyes, at the base of the upper and lower lashes. She wears a golden-tinted foundation and lots of warm-colored blusher on the cheekbones to make her face appear rounder. (Although she does like cool colors on her eyes and lips, she never uses them in her foundation or blusher.) Finally, to soften the total effect

even more, Carrie defines and colors her lips to make them slightly pouty.

Another Sagittarian beauty, model Carol Alt, also opts for a natural look when doing her own makeup. A clear, glossy shine under her eyes draws attention to them, lots of black mascara frames them, and a pale pink lip gloss completes her look.

The beautiful open smiles of Laura Antonelli and Jane Fonda soften the long angles and square brows of their faces. Both have learned through experience that their fine features are best enhanced with less rather than more. Jane Fonda, most notably, has come a long way since her earlier acting days. The vitality and natural, healthy good looks so obvious in her recent films are what Sagittarian beauty is all about.

c a p r i c o r n
d e c e m b e r   2 2 – j a n u a r y   2 0

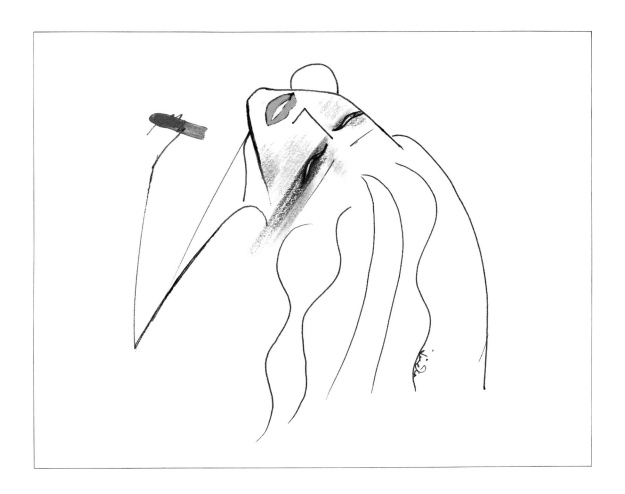

 When I think of the Capricorn woman, I immediately think of beautifully melancholy, captivating eyes. Their intensity, which belies the aura of cool aloofness typical of her sign, makes them her most attractive feature—and the most important aspect of her makeup. They should be emphasized with strong, blended makeup in dark misty colors, such as navy blue, gray, solid brown, and, as with the other earth signs, dark grayish or bottle green. These colors should be applied heavily next to the lashes, completely surrounding the eyes, and to help space them, blended straight out. Do not sweep the color upward; this will only lengthen the already long face that Capricorn usually has. The eyes, most often brown and sometimes small and round in shape, can be enlarged with black or brown eyeliner. The line should be very thin at the inner corner and across two-thirds of the eyelid, then rather wide at the outer corner to modify the shape.

While the youthful Capricorn is generally unsure of herself and weighed down by limitations and responsibilities, she will find that life becomes richer for her as she

73

grows older. Women of this sign are outwardly calm, elegant, and gracious, with natural "class." They create their images carefully, and while they never spend simply for the pleasure of spending, quality is of great importance to them. Uninfluenced by the latest fashions, they buy little but always well, and tend to choose established brands of skin-care products and makeup.

Still, Capricorn often has difficulties knowing how to use makeup and as a result may avoid it completely. This is unfortunate, because Capricorn has a very discreet beauty which benefits greatly from the emphasis given by cosmetics. A strong makeup can easily be carried by women of this sign; if intelligently applied, it strengthens the impact of their personality, as well as the public image that's so important to them.

Saturn, the ruler of Capricorn, often bestows an olive tint to the complexion, which becomes more beautiful as she grows older. In youth, however, she is prone to either acne or, at the other extreme, dry, flaky skin and allergies. The sun, good general health, and a disciplined skin-care regime begun in adolescence are essential to her skin's health. Capricorns should use cleansers instead of soaps and apply protective moisturizing creams daily. The fragile skin around the eyes profits from regular compresses of witch hazel and a very light eye cream. Both are better with-

stood and more effective in the morning rather than at night.

Very little blusher is needed to bring life to the Capricorn complexion. If the skin is pale, a light dusting of an almost white powder will make an extraordinary difference. If the makeup is too well balanced, it will be very boring on Capricorn, unless very unusual colors are used. On the other hand, too colorful or "trendy" a makeup will be overpowering to her subtle beauty.

The Capricorn woman generally has a rather small but beautifully shaped mouth. If the emphasis is here, she should first define the lips with a pencil of the same shade as the lipstick. Since the outline of her lips is not very strong, it is easy to enlarge the mouth if so desired. The lip color should then be taken completely to the pencil line. Bright red lipstick is flattering, but in that case the eye makeup should be discreet, or even nonexistent. If the eye makeup is strong, the lips should then be underplayed with light muted tones of pink or orange.

Capricorn is at her best wearing jet jewelry set in silver, with smoky-gray eye colors and bright red lipstick to add drama. Dark sapphires—another Capricorn stone—should be worn with a pale, muted lipstick, a minimum amount of blusher, and dark blue or gray on the eyes. Although slightly less dramatic, this look is just as effective in enhancing the elegance and magnetism of Capricorn's quiet beauty.

carol

To *modify*: The round eyes
The rather long face

To *accentuate*: The beautiful melancholy expression in the eyes
The distinguished elegance of Capricorn

74

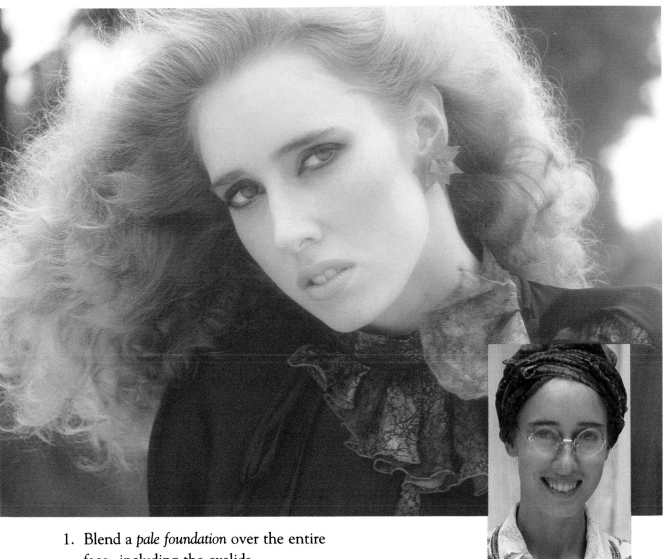

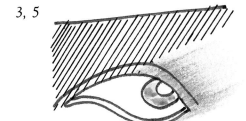

1. Blend a *pale foundation* over the entire face, including the eyelids.

2. Use a *medium gray pencil* at the base of the lashes—a little thicker in the upper outer corner—and on the bone just above the eye socket. This should be well blended a third of the way up to the eyebrows.

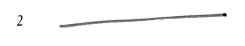

2

3. A *dark gray pencil* should then be applied next to the lashes in the upper outer corner. This too should be blended outward.

4. Powder the entire face, including the eyelids, with a *transparent face powder*.

3, 5

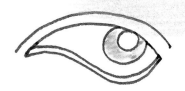

5. With a little *white powder eye shadow*, lighten the inner part of the eyelid and under the eyebrows.

6. Blend a *gray matte powder eye shadow* onto the outer part of the eyelid—the

75

part already shaded with the gray pencil—blending it outward.

7. Blend a *light tawny blusher* inward onto the cheek under the cheekbone. Care must be taken to take it straight across the face about halfway between the eye and the mouth to diminish the length. Taking the blusher down the face would lengthen it.

8. With a *white highlighter powder*, lighten the cheekbones to give them more fullness.

9. Accentuate the fullness of the lips with a *pale yellow-orange lipstick*.

7, 8

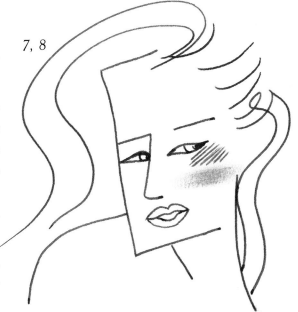

veronique

To modify: The dull skin
The round, rather close-set eyes
The size of the lips
To accentuate: The beautiful cheekbones
The intense "brunette" quality of the Capricorn beauty

1. A *very pale foundation* is first applied to the entire face, including the eyelids.

2. With a *dark navy kohl pencil*, completely color the mobile part of the eyelid, then under the bottom lashes, making sure that the base of the lashes is well covered. Blend outward.

3. Powder the whole face, including the eyelids, with a *transparent powder*.

4. Blend a *pale muted frosted pink powder eye shadow* on the eyelid next to the nose, then up and under the eyebrows.

5. Blend a *medium frosted brown powder eye shadow* from the outer corner of

the blue pencil shading upward and outward into the pale pink.

6. The navy-blue shading can then be reinforced if desired with a *dark blue frosted eye shadow.*

2, 4

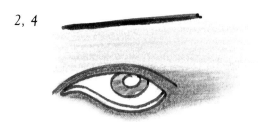

5, 7

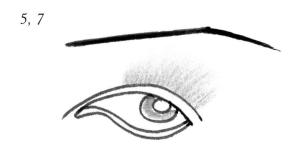

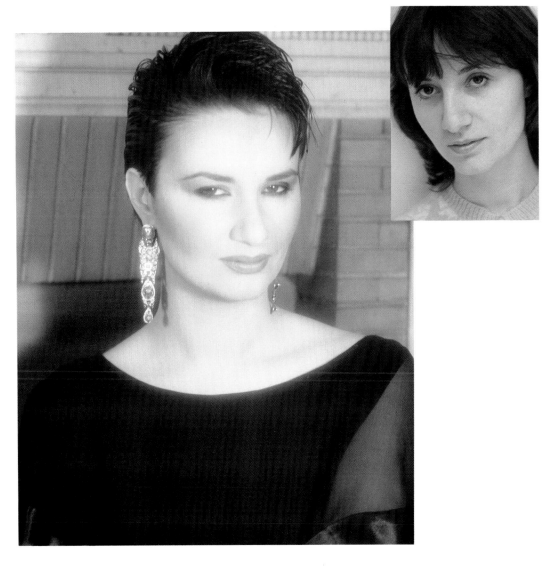

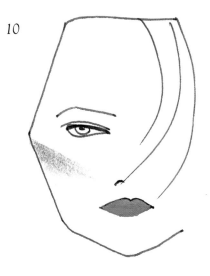

7. Apply a little *brown eyebrow pencil* to slightly lengthen the brows.

8. Apply *black mascara* to top and bottom lashes.

9. Line inside the lower rim of the eyes with a *black or dark blue kohl pencil.*

10. Use a little *muted pink blusher* just under the cheekbones.

11. Outline the mouth with a *muted pink lip pencil.* Make the line of the upper lip curved rather than straight by going outside the natural lip line as shown in the sketch. Enlarge the lower lip slightly to balance this.

12. With a lipbrush, fill in the lips with a *muted pale pink lipstick.*

10

11

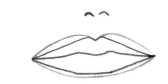

veronique (2)

To accentuate: The calm, practical Saturnian qualities of Capricorn

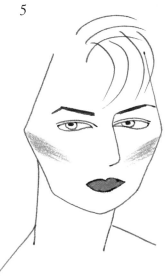

5

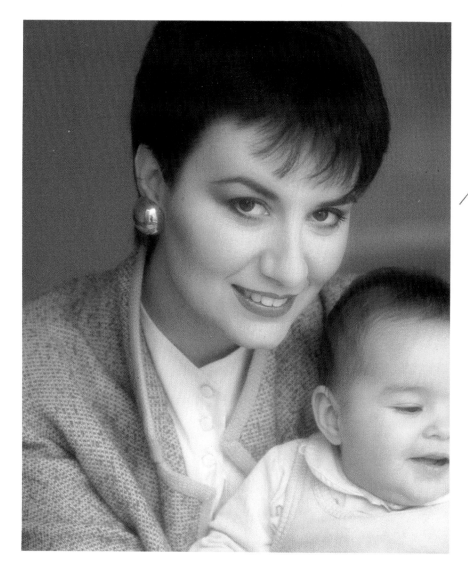

1. After applying base and powder as in Steps 1 and 3 of the previous makeover, apply a *brown powder eye shadow* to the mobile part of the eyelids and blend outward.

2. Blend a *matte pink eye shadow* under the eyebrows into the brown.

3. Accentuate the base of the bottom lashes with a *brown pencil*.

4. Use a *tawny blusher* low on the cheekbone, blending it inward onto the cheek.

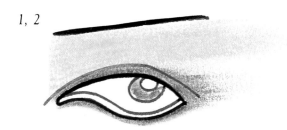

1, 2

5. With a *red pencil*, outline the lips, following the natural line.

6. Apply a *bright red lipstick* with a lipbrush.

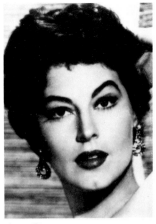

AVA GARDNER

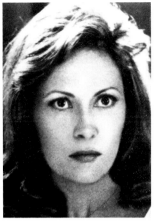

FAYE DUNAWAY

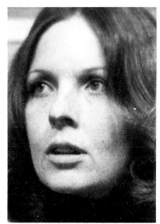

DIANE KEATON

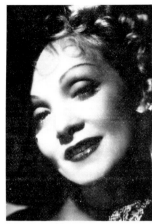

MARLENE DIETRICH

The peoples of India descend from an ancient tradition which, unlike that of the West, has remained alive and virtually unchanged after thousands of years. As their philosophy has remained the same, so has the beauty and makeup of the Hindu woman. She is strongly influenced by Capricorn both in facial characteristics and in the emphasis of her eyes. Like the modern Capricorn woman, she has found little need to experiment, having discovered the makeup that strengthens the impact of her appearance in the most effective way.

Marlene Dietrich is a perfect example of the Capricorn woman whose public image was shaped with the help of makeup. She enhanced her aloof, melancholy mystique by removing her sparse eyebrows and penciling them in, and applying heavy false eyelashes to the upper lid and white pencil inside the rim of the eye. Her beautiful cheekbones—another fairly typical Capricorn feature—were emphasized with shading under the cheekbone, rather than blusher.

Faye Dunaway was expertly transformed for her portrayal of Joan Crawford (Aries) in *Mommie Dearest*, but was betrayed by her melancholy Capricorn eyes. Faye is at her most beautiful when her face and lips

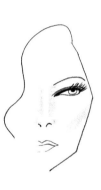

are kept natural and the emphasis is on her eyes: no color on the eyelids, but with the base of the upper lashes darkened; plenty of mascara; and false eyelashes in the upper outer corner of the eyes. Brown shading from the inner corner of the eyebrows down the sides of the nose gives more depth to this region.

French fashion designer Claude Montana (Cancer), whose clothes have a beautifully strong and rather dramatic look, feels that the most important makeup for him has *le glow dans la vie*—that is, the glow that emerges from the personality. Unsurprisingly, this is one of the most memorable qualities of his ideal beauty, Ava Gardner. Her rich, dark coloring, strong classic bone structure, and cat-like green eyes combine to produce that magnetism which is so uniquely hers.

Diane Keaton's aura of aloofness and haunting, melancholy eyes are another excellent example of Capricorn features. Although it would be easy to imagine her in Dietrich-style makeup, she has never used cosmetics as a tool to strengthen her image. Instead, her personal style and the wit and confidence she has brought to her films have created her successful and intriguing public image.

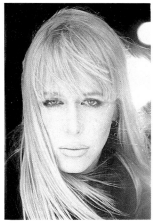 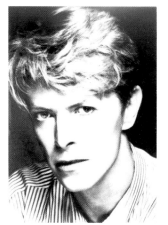

TERI TOYE   DAVID BOWIE

It is interesting to note that many pop stars are born under the sign of Capricorn and are generally very discreet in their makeup. An exception is David Bowie, who frequently uses makeup in a very strong way to reinforce his image. At one point, he wore foundation and shortened the length of his face by applying blusher under the cheekbone (as in Carol's makeover in this chapter). He darkened his eyes at the base of the upper and lower lashes and occasionally lengthened them by blending a light brown shadow outward (in the same way as the gray applied to Carol) and a light gray kohl pencil inside the lower rim. Note also his resemblance to model Teri Toye, who has developed a comfortable makeup for herself and, true to Capricorn style, rarely varies. Her makeup is also similar to that used in Carol's makeover in this chapter. Teri enlarges her dark green eyes by shading the base of the bottom lashes and the eye socket with gray, and by lightening the browbone. Her fine Capricorn eyebrows are hidden by her bangs; black eyeliner is applied to the base of the upper lashes, black kohl is used inside the lower rim of the eyes, and lots of black mascara is worn. Teri applies blusher in the same way as Carol and David Bowie—straight across the face under the cheekbones. By defining and enlarging her lips with a light brown pencil, then covering them with a light foundation, she attains a pale but fuller and more sensual effect for her typically Capricorn mouth.

aquarius

january 21 – february 19

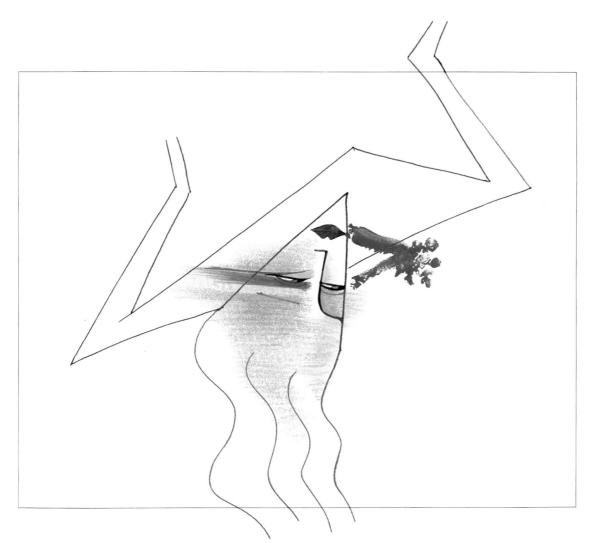

Aquarius women have an unusual touching quality. Haunting and wistful, they are among the most beautiful in the zodiac. They are always interesting-looking, with delicately chiseled features, and usually have blond or sandy-colored hair and a complexion paler than average within their ethnic group. The typical Aquarian face is long and triangular, with the base of the triangle at the forehead. The mouth is at one extreme or the other: thin lips, not well defined, with the upper lip thinner than the lower; or large, full, and rather elastic. The former generally accompanies a somewhat detached personality; the latter is found with larger, rounder faces and more exuberant personalities. The eyes are usually round, and although not drooping, they sometimes appear to dip because of the sharp downturn of the eyebrow bone in the center. The eyebrows are fine and usually straight.

Although Aquarius is never overly preoccupied with her appearance, she often ends up looking quite avant-garde. She is ready to try any type of skin treatment or makeup because she is capable of seeing herself objectively, with a certain curiosity. She also has a great love of color. This does not mean, however, that she herself enjoys experimenting; she would rather see what others can do for her. Because of this, Aquarius is the perfect model for the makeup artist: she's calm and confident enough to accept any new look.

Even if the Aquarius woman does not have the particular eye shape mentioned above, her eyes will probably be unusually shaped. That, combined with her long face, makes her makeup rather difficult. It must be kept light, and airy colors used. Grayish-browns are better than reddish hues, unless the hair is sandy-colored, and all shading must be well blended. Still, Aquarius can take a stronger and more unusual makeup well. She's at her best when experimenting and emphasizing her own originality. The more sensual, rounder-faced Aquarian, for example, can go with her oddly shaped eyes rather than against them, perhaps by highlighting the prominent part of the eyelids and darkening the deep crease in the inner corner. Color under the eyes also works well, unusual kohl colors inside the lower rim being but one possibility.

As with other air signs, a matte finish is best for Aquarian face powders and eye shadows, to enhance the beauty of her naturally pale skin. The most flattering eye colors are pastels; mustard, violet, and all shades of gray, especially grayish-blues. Blusher should be placed on the cheekbone of the narrower-faced Aquarius—if placed under the cheek it will only lengthen and slim the face even more. Light or muted pinks and light peaches are best for this. On her lips, all bluish tints look good, from pale bluish-pink through lilac and on to violet. For those with thicker lips, pale muted lipsticks and transparent glosses are most attractive.

When Uranus, the ruler of Aquarius, is strong, amber jewelry will add warmth and offer an unusual and flattering contrast to her bluish shades of makeup. This is especially becoming to sandy-haired, freckle-faced Aquarians. When Saturn, the co-ruler, is strong, the skin tends to be sallower. In this case, sapphire or black pearls, also associated with Aquarius, will be more flattering, and will harmonize beautifully with all shades of lilac, deep violet, or gray on the eyes and muted pink on the lips.

paula

To modify: The sunken eyes
The roundness of the face and eyes

To accentuate: The sensual lips
The haunting wistfulness of the Aquarian

1. A *pale shade of foundation* should be applied to the whole of the face, including the eyelids.

2. Blend into the under-eye area and lids a *paler and thicker foundation or concealer.*

3. Apply a *creamy peach eye shadow* to the mobile part of the eyelid.

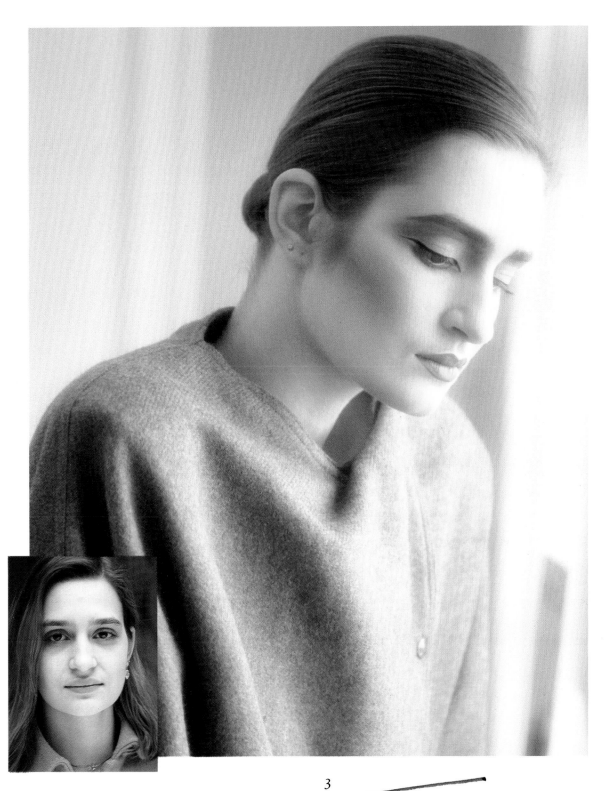

4. Outline the lips with a *garnet-colored pencil*, starting in the middle and working outward on both upper and lower lips. The line should be very fine in the corners of the mouth, and blended inward. Always support your head with the little finger of the hand with which you are working; the elbow of this arm should be supported

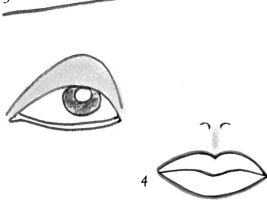

as well. The lips should be relaxed, and to blend and check the pencil line, it helps to smile.

5. With a *white pencil*, outline the garnet line and philtrum (the two lines running from the nostrils to the lips). Blend these lines with a fine brush (the garnet one inward and the white one outward).

6. Use a *transparent powder* to powder the entire face, including the eyelids and lips.

7. A *brown matte powder eye shadow or blusher* should be applied from the inner part of the eyebrow, blended across the eyebrow bone and straight out, then lightly down the sides of the nose from the eyebrows. A touch should also be applied in the philtrum, and more under the cheekbones, stronger on the outer edge of the face, then blended inward and down.

8. Apply a *pale turquoise pencil* inside the lower rim of the eye, extending it inward toward the nose and straight out in the outer corner for about ⅛″. If you cannot find pale turquoise, mix white with a darker one. Blend it well into the lashes, and a little down under the eye.

7

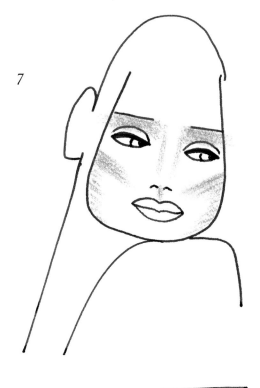

8

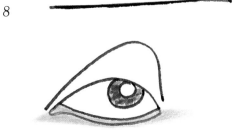

10, 11

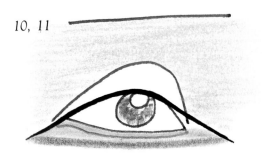

14

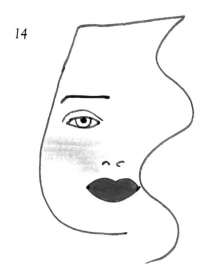

9. With a *peach-colored powder eye shadow*, reinforce the already colored eyelid.

10. With a *black liquid eyeliner*, trace a very fine line at the base of the upper lashes, starting at the innermost corner and finishing at the end of the pale turquoise pencil.

11. With a *navy blue powder eye shadow* on a small brush, very delicately shade

under the turquoise from the inner to the outer corners. This should join the end of the black liner.

12. With a *light brown pencil*, make the eyebrows a little longer and more angular. With this type of makeup it is important that the eyebrows be well defined.

13. Apply *black mascara* to the upper lashes.

14. Apply a *peach-colored powder blusher* to the cheeks, blending it into the brown.

15. A *light-colored muted pink lipstick* should then be used on the lips. Take care not to hide the lip line completely.

vanessa

To modify: The rather long forehead
The round eyes, deep-set and close together
The long, narrow face

To accentuate: The blueness of the eyes
The naturally tranquil Aquarian nature

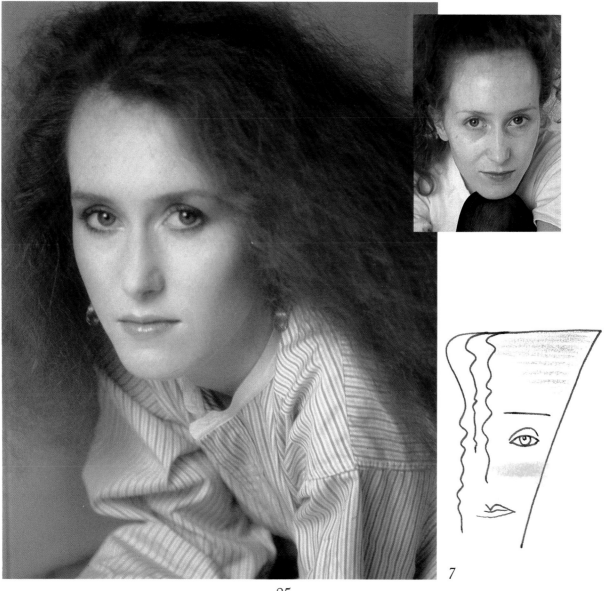

7

85

1. A *very pale, almost white under-eye concealer* should first be used in the upper inner corners of the eye and in the under-eye area.

2. Next, a *very pale foundation* should be used over the entire face, and blended well with the under-eye cream.

3. Under the eyes, a little heavier in the outer corner, and in the outer part of the socket, apply a *russet pencil or eye shadow.* This will harmonize with the hair and set off the blue eyes. This shade should be blended out and upward to space the eyes.

4. Dust the entire face, including the eyelids, with a *transparent powder.*

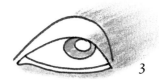 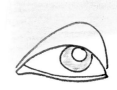

5. A *light shade of mustardy-beige matte eye shadow* should then be applied to the uncolored part of the eye and blended with the russet shading.

6. Lightly color the eyebrows with a *yellowish light brown pencil.*

7. Blend a *light pink blusher* into the center of the cheeks to give a fuller look to the face.

8. Apply a *pale pink semi-transparent lipstick* to the lips.

vanessa (2)

To accentuate: The Aquarian originality

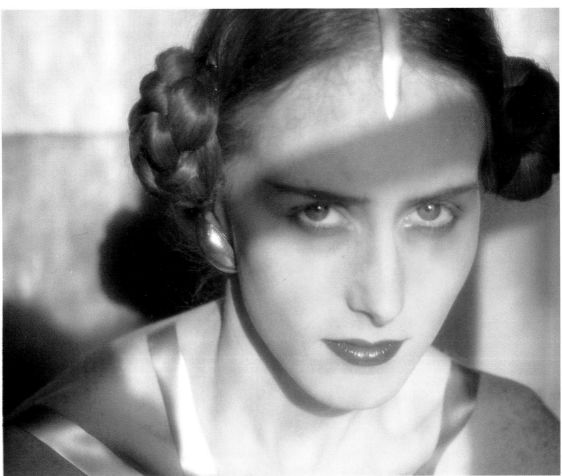

Perform Steps 1 and 2 as in the previous makeover.

3. Cover the upper lid of one eye with a *pale blue cream eye shadow.* Blend outward.

4. Blend a *mustard cream eye shadow* under the bottom lashes of this same eye. Darken the base of the lashes further with a *russet-colored pencil.* Apply this same shadow on the other eye, to the inner half of the eye, both above and below, taking it to an imaginary line running down from the eyebrow through the center of the eye.

5. A *pink cream eye shadow* should then be blended around the outer part of this eye, from the lashes up to the eyebrow and down onto the cheekbone. Darken the base of the lashes with a *darker pink pencil* to give more depth.

6. Dust the entire face with a *transparent face powder,* taking special care when powdering the made-up eyes.

7. Use a *yellowish light brown pencil* to straighten and lengthen the eyebrows, drawing them straight out.

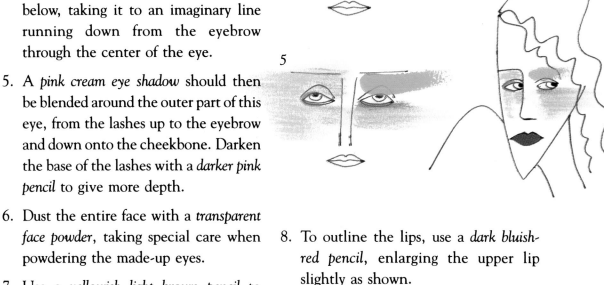

8. To outline the lips, use a *dark bluish-red pencil,* enlarging the upper lip slightly as shown.

9. With a lipbrush, apply a *violet shade of lipstick.*

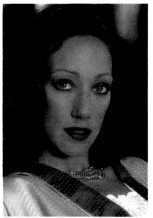

MARISA BERENSON

Marisa Berenson is a perfect example of the Aquarius with a long and triangular face. Her extremely pale skin and ethereal quality made her the perfect Countess of Lyndon in Stanley Kubrick's film *Barry Lyndon.* Marisa knows better than anyone how intense her eye makeup can be if she wants to lengthen and give depth to her beautiful blue eyes, in order to accentuate the more sensual side of her Aquarian nature. Dark misty blues and grays are perfect for this, as is the brown makeup used on Vanessa earlier in this chapter.

The influence of Uranus is stronger in the case of the rounder-faced, fuller-lipped Aquarian. Model and actress Maud Adams typifies this category. She uses an ivory-colored face wash to enhance the

87

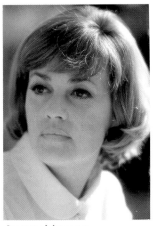

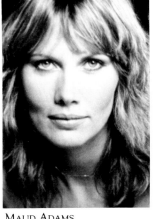

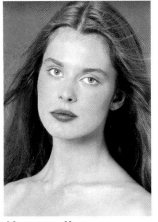

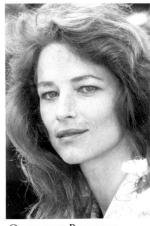

JEANNE MOREAU · MAUD ADAMS · NASTASSJA KINSKI · CHARLOTTE RAMPLING

translucence of her skin. Since her cheekbones are full and rounded, she looks very good without blusher but will usually use it in a natural tone to give her cheeks a healthy glow. Often, Maud lengthens her eyes and accentuates the base of the bottom lashes with gray pencil. She likes shades of gray in her eye makeup, or earth tones mixed with a light violet. When she appears on television, her makeup artist uses a dark bluish-gray liquid eyeliner, sometimes mixed with a gray pencil to soften the line, to reinforce the brilliance of her blue Aquarian eyes. Her sparse eyebrows are thickened slightly with a very light golden-beige eyebrow pencil, and her full lips defined with a light pinkish-brown pencil. Usually she wears a muted pink lipstick with a more bluish-pink lip gloss on top.

In the same category as Maud Adams are the stunning actresses Jeanne Moreau and Nastassja Kinski. Their facial structures are startlingly similar, but more important is the aura which all these women share. Their beauty is haunting and feminine, yet at the same time there is an independence of spirit which shines through.

The beautiful Aquarian Charlotte Rampling has the unusual but very attractive hooded eyes that are often found under this sign (and under Pisces). I find this shape lends an intense, distant, "untouch-

able" quality to the face. Many women with these eyes complain that they are difficult to make up. But not only is this type of eye just as beautiful without makeup (since the expression is just as strong), there are also, contrary to belief, many ways of making it up.

To exaggerate the overhanging lid, one could blend a pale lavender, or any extremely pale, unusual shade, over the entire lid to the eyebrows. This should not be an iridescent shadow, but a chalky matte or creamy one.

To lift the lid a bit and open the eye, use a medium brown shadow in a neutral tone from the inner eyelid near the nose, carry over the fold, and blend outward. Then use a highlighter on the spot just under the apex of the eyebrow, as shown in the sketch.

To lengthen the eye, and at the same time lift the lid slightly, brown shading in the outer corner blended up and outward from the base of the upper lashes will do the trick.

For a stronger effect with any of these makeups, the base of the bottom lashes could be darkened slightly with a soft grayish-brown pencil, and brown mascara applied. Eyeliner, although it will be covered wholly or partially by the fold of skin, is good for this eye, as it reinforces color at the base of the lashes and can be extended at the outer corner to lengthen the shape.

p i s c e s

february 20 – march 20

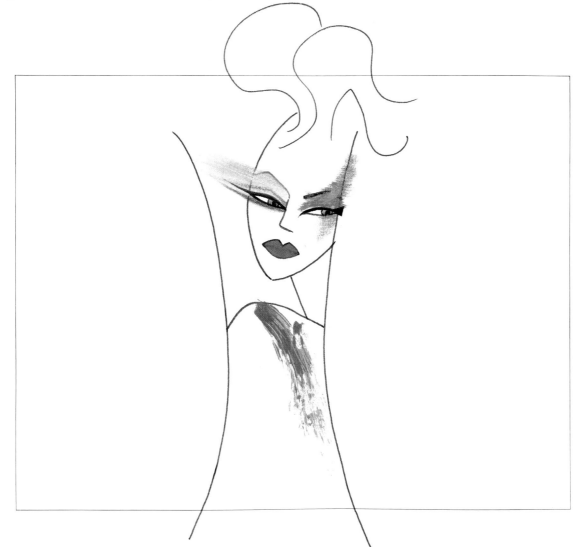

Pisces is a true water sign: fluid, poetic, and feminine. She is the luminous, ethereal mermaid with the beautifully rounded figure, melting, watery eyes in a compelling face, and a vulnerability that makes one long to protect her. Pisces is easily moved to tears—of joy as well as sorrow—so if she has any beauty problem at all, it will probably be with her eyes. They are usually quite large and protruding, with a tendency to swell. They can be soothed very nicely, however, with compresses of witch hazel.

The Piscean face is most often oval-shaped, with a rounded forehead and strong, radiant skin that will remain smooth and silky until comparatively late in life if she protects it from the sun. Because of the uniformity of her skin tone, her wonderfully balanced features, her beautiful, often unusual eye color (watery green, transparent blue, or violet), and the mobility of her face, Pisces is one sign that has little physical need for makeup. Her fragility and a certain shyness, however, give her a strong psychological need for it. She can be carried away by the vast array of beauty products available, and her

89

shyness and vulnerability make her an easy prey for avid salesclerks. What she should remember above all is to respect the harmony of her features by using makeup of uniform intensity—whatever overall effect she desires.

No foundation will be needed for the natural look, but she should apply a moisturizer to protect her skin and a dusting of fine powder down the center of her face. The powder could be opalescent, as a slight shine is especially attractive on Pisces.

The space between her eyes and eyebrows is generally quite open and can be covered with shadow, but a darker color should be used next to the lashes to give her eyes more depth. Their oblique, almond shape can be accentuated with silvery-gray, gray-blue, gray-green, or even turquoise liner. Black eyeliner will harden her soft expression, but if a more dramatic effect is desired, it can certainly be used. The smoothness of the Piscean eyelid

makes it quite easy to apply the frosted shadows which are so flattering to her limpid eyes. The most beautiful eye colors for her are those associated with her ruling planet, Neptune—lavender, mauve, sea-green, and aquamarine—all ethereal shades. While these colors can be harsh and detrimental to other signs, they acquire a wonderful softness and tranquillity on the eternally fresh and youthful Piscean complexion.

Appropriately, coral jewelry is the most becoming to Pisces, especially when worn with the bluer shades of pink or red lipstick that look so good on her, and with eyes discreetly colored with smoky gray (another Neptune color) or dark deep-sea blue. Another Piscean stone, the amethyst, can be worn to enhance the effect of lilac eye shadow and lipstick, or to contrast with sea-green eye color—either would be especially beguiling on this sparkling water sign.

chandrika

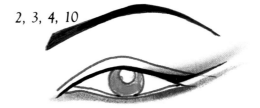

2, 3, 4, 10

To modify: The rather small mouth
   The color of the skin
To accentuate: The eyes, eyebrows, and
   cheekbones
   The dramatic side of Pisces'
   nature

1. The skin is lightened with a *heavy foundation* much lighter in tone than the complexion. This is mainly an evening makeup; in the daytime this color change would be too obvious.

If the skin is tanned, it will be more difficult to cover. First soften the face by massaging with almond oil, as the skin must be supple. If the foundation is not heavy enough, the skin will soon show through in patches, making the aspect gray and blotchy.

2. With a *white pencil,* apply a very fine line in the outer corner of the eyes. Start above the actual corner to lift the line a little, and follow the natural

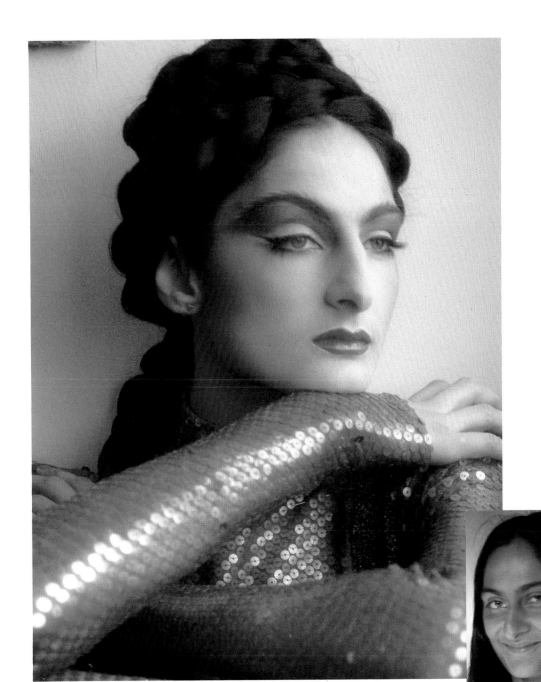

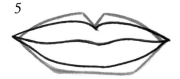

sweep of the eyes so that the uplift is not too abrupt.

3. Blend a little *burgundy pencil* above the white, taking it outward to emphasize this lift.

4. At the base of the bottom lashes, blend a little *violet pencil.*

5. With a *dark red pencil*, outline the lips. Begin by enlarging the center of the lips as shown, making them slightly larger and squarer. Then gradually complete the line until you have the shape you desire.

5

6. With a finely sharpened *white pencil* or white foundation on a fine brush, outline the dark red pencil.

7. Dust the entire face, including the eyelids and lips, with a very heavy, pale, and opaque *face powder.* This fixes the pencil shading so it will not run.

91

8. Apply a *pale shimmery-pink powder eye shadow or blusher* to the mobile part of the eyelid. Apply this same pink high on the cheekbone, next to the violet.

9. A *sea-green powder eye shadow with iridescent bronze highlights* should then be applied under the eyebrow over the browbone, blending outward.

10. Apply a very fine line of *black eyeliner* next to the upper lashes, extending above the white line in the outer corner of the eyes.

11. Apply *black mascara* to upper and lower lashes.

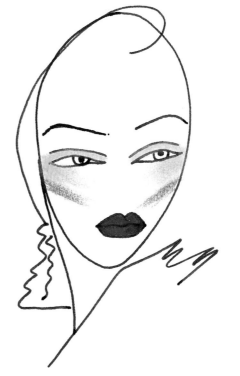

9

12. On the liner at the outer corner of the eye, apply about four clusters of *false eyelashes*—two next to the eye and two following the upward sweep, gradually becoming longer.

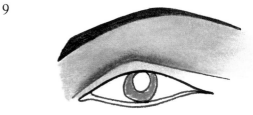

13. Under the outer corner of the lower lid, apply about three very short clusters of lashes, the longer ones at the outer corner.

12, 13, 14

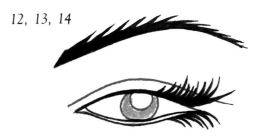

14. Brush the eyebrows upward. Alternating a sharp *dark reddish- or grayish-brown with a white pencil*, apply light strokes to the brows to exaggerate their shape and size. Apply an extremely fine white line under the eyebrows.

15. Apply *white pencil* inside the lower rim of the eyes.

16. Under the cheekbone, apply a sweep of *dark bluish-red powder blusher*. Blend downward toward the corners of the mouth.

17. With a lipbrush, apply a *ruby-colored lipstick*.

birgit

To *modify*: The slightly protruding eyes
To *accentuate*: The harmony of the features
The upward sweep of the eyes
The smoothness of the skin

1. Apply a *pale transparent foundation* to the entire face, including the eyelids.

2. Shade the mobile part of the eyelids with *dark blue pencil*, blending up and outward to follow the sweep of the eyes. Keep the color more intense next to the lashes. Apply a little of this same color to the base of the bottom lashes.

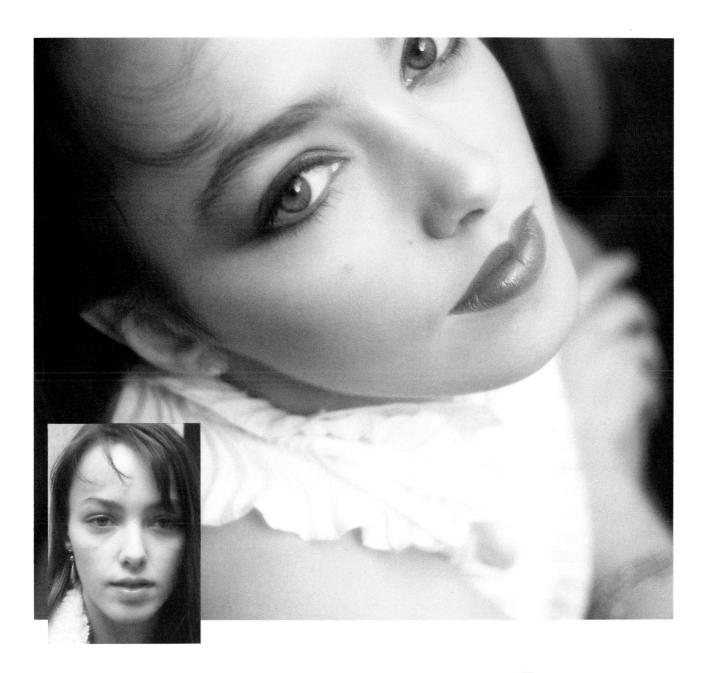

3. With a *transparent powder*, dust the entire face, including the eyelids.

4. Apply a *frosted cream-colored powder eye shadow* from the blue pencil to the eyebrows.

5. Apply a *dark blue frosted eye shadow* on top of the blue pencil and blend it into the cream coloring.

6. The blue shadow will become yellower when blended into the cream. This can be emphasized by applying a bit of *frosted turquoise* to this part of the eye.

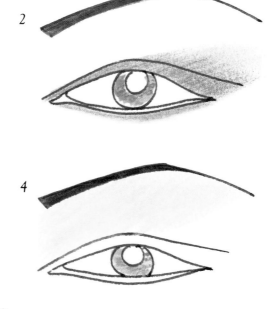

93

7. A *dark blue liquid eyeliner* is then applied to the base of the upper lashes following the upward tilt of the eyes.

8. Apply *blue mascara* to upper and lower lashes.

9. Line inside the rim of the lower lashes with a *turquoise kohl* pencil.

10. A *light bluish-pink powder blusher* is then applied to the cheekbone and blended down into the center of the cheeks.

11. For a shiny, dewy look, powder the face lightly with an *opalescent transparent powder*.

12. Apply a *bluish-pink shade of lipstick*.

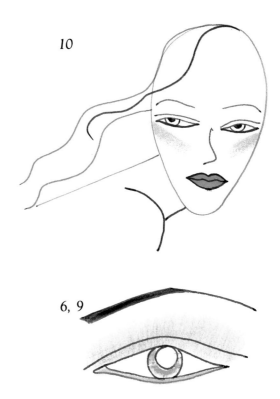

10

6, 9

mary rita

To *modify*: The rather swollen under-eye area

To *accentuate*: The soft femininity of the Piscean woman

1. Apply a *very pale foundation* to the entire face.

2. With a brush, apply a little *white foundation*, mixed with pale foundation, to the deep line beneath the swollen under-eye area.

3. Dab the Piscean *turquoise and green cream eye shadow* asymmetrically onto the eyelids with the fingers. Put more of the darker color nearer the eyes.

4. These two rather cool colors should be warmed up on the redhead with a touch of *orange cream eye shadow* at the inner and outer corners of the eyes.

5. A little *off-white highlighter* should then be dotted into this mixture.

6. Mix *transparent and white face powder* and dust the entire face, including the eyelids.

7. The cream shadows on the eyelids can be strengthened by pressing *turquoise and green powder shadows* over them with the fingers.

8. With the *palest bluish-pink powder blusher*, color the center of the cheeks.

9. Color two-thirds of the upper lip with a *pale bluish-pink pencil*, and the remaining third with an *apricot pencil*. Then color two-thirds of the lower lip with the apricot pencil and the remaining third with the pink pencil. To facilitate this, first apply lip gloss, then wipe it off. This will leave the lips slightly greasy and clean them of foundation at the same time. Blend the pencil with a lipbrush.

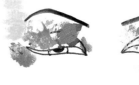

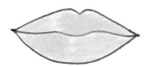

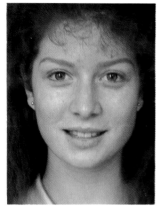

8

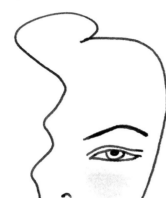

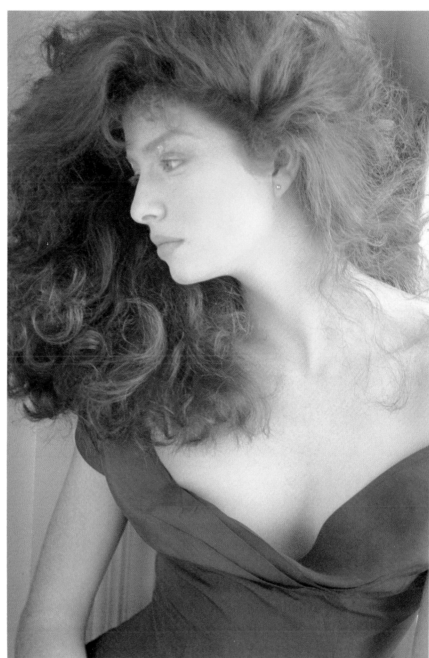

Rapturously beautiful Elizabeth Taylor has every attribute of the perfect Piscean woman, the most outstanding, of course, being her famous eyes. Francesco Scavullo (Capricorn) has said that Ms. Taylor is brilliant in every aspect of her makeup, including the violet-blue eye shadow which brings out the violet in her eyes. (Bronze or green shadow would have this same wonderful effect.) She rarely needs blusher; her gleaming skin and soft oval face are qualities that made Richard Burton prefer her without makeup. It is truly remarkable how little her complexion has changed since her youth.

Ms. Taylor is very adept at lining her eyes to further accentuate their phenomenal color and shape. To apply eyeliner in a smooth and professional way, turn your head down and to the left, and apply to the inner corner of the left eye and the outer part of the right (fig. a). Turn your

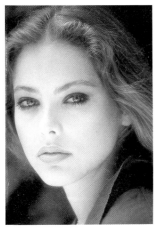

ORNELLA MUTTI

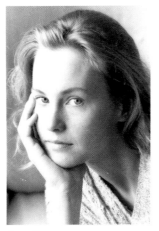

LISE RYALL

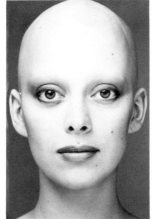

JENNY-O

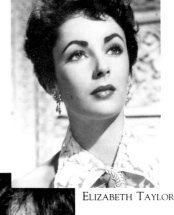

ELIZABETH TAYLOR

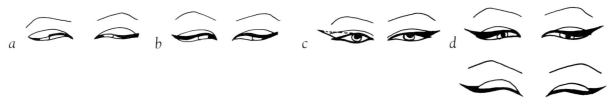

head down and to the right and apply to the inner corner of the right eye and the outer part of the left (fig. b). Look straight ahead and relax your eye and eyebrow muscles completely to avoid distorting the line. Lengthen the line with the eyes wide open (fig. c), starting slightly above the outer corner of the eye. Fill in the liner from the outermost corner of the line to the center (fig. d). The line should be very fine in the inner corner and widened slightly at the outer corner. It is most important that the liner look smooth when the eyes are open, so fight the temptation to close them when filling in the line. Then lift your head and check with the eyes lowered.

The similarity between the two Piscean actresses Ornella Mutti and Lise Ryall is astonishing. When Lise wears makeup, she prefers her face to be matte and white, with no blusher, and enhances her delicate features with pale eye colors such as iridescent green or pale orange. Her lips are stained rather than painted: to do this,

you can rub on a little lip pencil, then blend with your finger. Alternatively, you can apply a rather heavy wine-colored lipstick (Lise's favorite color for winter), blot several times, rub with your finger, and then powder. If you have dry lips, apply lip gloss and blot before applying the lipstick.

Model Jenny-O enjoys makeup, and for her very pale skin uses an ivory foundation with a translucent powder. She never wears mascara; instead, she lines her eyes inside and out with gray or purple eye pencil for intensity, and gives them depth by using powder shadows in purples, browns, or pinks. She takes great care of her luminous skin—in her photograph you can see immediately the soft, oval face and perfectly balanced features of the Piscean woman.

Index

Brown to black hair—one shade lighter than the hair color
Darker redhead—a medium reddish-brown
Lighter redhead—a light mustardy brown
Blond—start with a gold pencil, then work in a light brown
Gray to silver hair—a mixture of gray and silver pencils

For a more realistic effect, it is almost always advisable to use a mixture of two colors. If you are still not quite sure of the best shades for your brows, start with gold and gradually darken the color.

When eyeliner is used, eyebrows usually need darkening. If the cheeks are sunken, then lightening the eyebrows will counteract that effect.

A touch of rouge on the bone just beneath the eyebrow or a dot of rouge at the tear duct will add a youthful sparkle. This is a common trick used with theatrical makeup, but can be adapted for ordinary cosmetics.

eyebrows

If the shape is not too drooping, they are very beautiful left natural on young girls. On the mature woman they are usually more flattering if lightly plucked. Before plucking, brush the eyebrows, then draw in the desired shape. For a natural shape, start sketching the brows on a line which is directly over the inner corner of the eye, continuing in upward, outward strokes. Color the natural hair or sketch the hair on the skin with fine hair-like lines if the brow is too thin or plucked in certain areas. The apex should be in line with the outer curve of the iris of the eye, and from this point the brow should curve down with the strokes still going outward. The tapered end of the brows should be about half an inch from the outer corner of the eye, as shown in the sketch, p. 15.

To tweeze, stretch the area of the skin where the eyebrows are to be plucked between the forefinger and the middle finger of one hand, then with the tweezers in the other hand pull the hairs out in the direction of their growth. Never pluck the eyebrows above their natural line.

eyelashes

If straight, they can be gently curled with eyelash curlers before applying mascara. Dyeing is best for thick eyelashes, as thin ones will only look more sparse and artificial when accentuated with color. Fair eyelashes are often very attractive left as they are, to give a soft, unusual look to the eye, as on p. 60, 94. This is especially becoming to the water signs. When doing a natural makeup, take care not to darken the lashes too much. Light brown for a light redhead, dark brown for a dark redhead or a blonde (or brunette, for a softer look), and black for a normal makeup on a brunette are the most suitable colors.

eyeliner

Can be liquid or cake, whichever you prefer. The brush you use is the most important factor in applying it. It should be fine sable, and not too long or soft. There are very good automatic liners on the market with perfectly adequate brushes; p. 3, 5, 8, 13, 18, 23, 31, 38, 46, 47, 53, 55, 66, 71, 84, 88, 92, 94, 96.

eyes

Blue, p. 2, 12, 20, 27, 35, 36, 43, 60, 95; green, p. 91, 93; brown, p. 4, 6, 11, 29, 44; hazel, p. 19, 21, 30, 52; protruding, p. 43; drooping, p. 50; deep-set, p. 29; close-set (less than the width of an eye apart), p. 10; wide (more than the width of an eye apart), p. 27; small, p. 2, 27; round, p. 34; almond-shaped, p. 18; Oriental, p. 6; oblique, p. 18, 20, 21; hooded, p. 88.

eye shadows

Matte, p. 19, 41, 82; cream, p. 47, 54, 61, 67, 87; frosted, p. 25, 52, 69, 76, 90.

face shapes

Round, p. 27; square, p. 34; oval, p. 43; hexagonal or heart-shaped, p. 49, 77; rectangular, p. 17, 65; triangular, p. 17, 81; trapezoidal, p. 9, 83. These shapes can be modified greatly by hair style. This is why it is advisable to do one's makeup with the hair down, in its usual style, rather than drawn off the forehead.

facial tones

If positioned in the right place, certain uneven facial colorations can be attractive. If it happens to be the nose that is bright red, then, of course, this is best corrected; p. 34. To do a more sophisticated makeup where face-shaping is called for, it is advisable to even out the skin tone first. High color in a complexion can be corrected by a green-tinted moisturizer and a grayish shade of foundation. A too-sallow complexion is best made a little more ivory, beige, or golden. It should not, under normal circumstances, be made pink; p. 10.

false eyelashes

Are staging a comeback. They should be applied when the eye makeup is finished. They are more natural when applied in small clusters (p. 92) rather than a whole band. First, measure them to make sure they are not bigger than the actual eye. Then brush the base of the lashes with a light coat of eyelash adhesive, wait a moment, and apply the false lashes as close as possible to the natural lash line; p. 71.

fire signs

Aries, p. 1; Leo, p. 33; Sagittarius, p. 65.

forehead

How to diminish, p. 27, 61; to enlarge, p. 10.

foundation

Should be as close as possible to the natural skin color, which is usually that of the neck. By evening out the color of the face, you eliminate distracting tints, and the eyes and mouth immediately become more noticeable, able to be enhanced further with makeup. Foundation is also excellent protection against pollution, harmful light rays, and other environmental hazards. A lightweight foundation with good coverage is usually best for all women. If it is fairly liquid, then it is most easily applied with the hands. A denser type is applied with a damp sponge, or, for heavier coverage, with a dry sponge. The skin must be in perfect condition if you want to darken it with foundation; otherwise, blemishes will trap the dark pigment and be accentuated. Darkening can be done gradually, by first applying a light foundation, then a slightly darker one, then the shade required—making a rather heavy makeup. To lighten, p. 90.

freckles
Fortunately, they are now looked upon as an asset, but they are also a sign of fine, delicate skin that must be well cared for. A transparent foundation should be worn, or at most, a light application of one with more coverage. Blend under the eyes and down the center of the face so the freckles are not hidden; p. 34.

glasses
Makeup should be strengthened when glasses are worn. Blusher should be applied with the glasses on, as the intensity and shape are easier to determine. If your glasses have colored rims, remember that this could influence the choice of colors in your makeup. Choose the frames for your glasses while wearing no makeup. If the color alone enhances your face, they are the best for you.

gold

gray

green

hair
Do not forget that you should not only try out new makeup colors to match a new hair color, but you can try new hair colors to suit your makeup. Your hair and makeup should become one. Cancer women enjoy being redheads, while Geminis and Leos often become blond.

highlighters

lip gloss
Good for natural protection while giving the lips a transparent shine, or touch of color, and a rich, healthy appearance. Although it is thought of as a modern innovation, perfumed lip salves were being sold even at the turn of the century.

lip pencils
It is best if the lip pencil is soft and well sharpened. The darker and more definite the lip outline, the more sophisticated the makeup becomes. To draw the lips as naturally as possible, choose a pencil the color of your lips or slightly lighter. In most cases a muted brownish-pink is good. Blend it well with a brush or your finger, then powder the pencil to fix it and keep it from smudging.

lips
Correction for, p. 5, 28, 30, 35, 37, 51, 71, 77. Do not forget that even a fraction of an inch added to the lips can make an enormous difference. If you study your lips carefully, you will probably find a darker red lip line, then, a little farther out, a lighter line, which is the rim of the lips. For natural enlargement, define this outer edge well, unless it is flat and undefined, in which case you can go a little farther. By coloring only as far as the inner line, or by not defining well at all, you can make your lips appear a little smaller. If the shape needs altering, cover the edge first with foundation. Marilyn Monroe's, p. 23.

lipstick
Is more natural if used without lip pencil. Make sure the lips are free of foundation and powder before applying lipstick. If the lips have been lined with a pencil, start applying the lipstick from the center of the lips, tapering off to the edges. To prevent running, do not take it right to the edge. Then blot.

mascara
To thicken the lashes well, first use a rather dry mascara with a thick brush. Then build up the mascara in layers with a wetter, creamier one. To keep the lashes separate—and really get to the base of them—move the brush from side to side when going from the base to the tips, let dry in between applications, and comb with a small eyelash comb. This is especially necessary with fair lashes, to make them blend in well with the rest of the eye makeup.

neck
To slim, p. 10, 30.

nose
Narrowing the width, p. 22, 37; highlighting, p. 28. To shorten a long, narrow nose, the under-eye area and the sides of the nose should be lightened considerably to space the eyes. If the nose is wide as well, then the same area should be lightened, but at the top the sides of the nose should be slightly darkened; p. 37.

orange

Oriental women, makeup for

pale skin
Beautiful to set off color, but colors should be used more delicately than on darker skins, as they will have more impact; p. 8, 60, 95.

pink

powder
Powder should be light in weight, have little or no color, and never streak or build up. If not transparent, it should always be lighter than the foundation color, to avoid thickening the skin. It is best applied with a cotton puff and pressed lightly into the foundation, as cotton wool leaves fluff and does not hold the powder so well. Do not pull the puff over the skin, as this could disturb the foundation. Lilac powder whitens the skin.

purple

red

redheads

rictus
Sometimes very deep lines appear from the sides of the nose to the outer corners of the mouth (at the rictus muscles). These can be alleviated by a good nourishing cream and a few facial exercises. If the makeup tends to collect here, rub lightly with a little almond oil, then reapply a little pale foundation and powder.

scars

If small, they can usually be hidden in the same way as blemishes. If deep, they can be filled in either with a thick cream foundation, or, if this is not enough, a little nose putty (found in theatrical shops). Blend putty into and over the scar, then cover with concealer.

shading

To correct the shape of the nasal bridge, p. 37; to minimize the forehead, p. 27, 61; to correct eye spacing, p. 10, 27, 29; to shade under the chin, p. 30; for a double chin, p. 30.

storage

Are you a hoarder? Do you have drawers full of used makeup products? Then make yourself an artist's palette for your dresser. Buy a cardboard artist's folder (preferably a small one). Remove all your eye shadows and blushers from their boxes by prying them out with a pin or heating in the oven to melt the plastic boxes. If this does not work, simply remove their lids. Arrange them on the folder in an attractive way, then glue them down. Keep them clean by covering with kitchen wrap.

utensils

These should be washed in warm, soapy water and rinsed well as often as possible. This is not only good hygiene but makes application of makeup smoother as well. Sable hair is usually the softest for eye shadow and blusher brushes. The sponge-tipped applicator is often better for the creamier powder shadows and flakier frosted ones, since more pressure is needed in applying them and they tend to fly all over the face if applied with a brush. The length of the brush is important, as this controls the flexibility; thus, the hairs should not extend too far. This is especially important to bear in mind when choosing a lipbrush.

water signs

Cancer, p. 25; Scorpio, p. 57; Pisces, p. 89.

white

p. 7.

yellow

p. 18.

The author extends heartfelt thanks to the models, hairdressers, stylists, and designers named below:

Aries: Lilo Zinglerson: hair, Melodie; clothing, Jean-Paul Gaultier. Ruth Gallardo: hair and clothing, Anthony Villareal. Noriko Tanaka: hair, Romain of Patrick Ales; clothing, Anne Marie Beretta.

Taurus: Deborah Barrett: hair, Mary Beth of Bumble & Bumble; clothing, Willi Wear. Geri Motto: hair, Regis of Bruno Dessange; clothing, Angelo Tarlazzi; picture #2, hair, Kyo; clothing, Nuit D'Elodie.

Gemini: Laure Killing: clothing, Guy Paulin; styling, Sylko. Veronica [Veroniqua] Chedal-Anglay: hair, Alexis. Caroline Fabre: hair, Kyo.

Cancer: Emilie [Evelyne] De Brauw: clothing, Jean-Paul Gaultier. Jody Pavlis: hair, Melodie. Melodie Lemaistre: hair, clothing, and styling by Linda Mason. African: Pierre Francillon.

Leo: Susan Scher: hair, clothing, and styling by Linda Mason. Katy Allen: hair, Mary Beth of Bumble & Bumble; picture #2, styling, Catherine Laroche.

Virgo: Tracy Leigh: hair, Anthony Villareal. Mariama [Danielle Cartillier]: clothing, Jean-Paul Gaultier; picture #2, hair, clothing, and styling by Linda Mason.

Libra: Cornelia Wilms: hair, Melodie; clothing, Anthony Villareal. Laura Gomez: hair, clothing, and styling by Linda Mason.

Scorpio: Patricia Barzyk: hair, Melodie; clothing, Anthony Villareal. Allyson Wacht: hair, Melodie.

Sagittarius: Barbara Thulin: hair, Odile of Bruno Dessange; clothing, Mary Jane Marcasiano; styling, Catherine Laroche. Lari Taylor: hair, Ezel of Bumble & Bumble; clothing, Anne Marie Beretta; turquoise jewelry by Jamie Simpson.

Capricorn: Carol Michelson: clothing, Bernard Danae. Veronique Courtoy: hair, Alexis.

Aquarius: Paula Spiaggia: clothing, Anne Marie Beretta. Vanessa Downing: hair, Melodie; styling, Sylko.

Pisces: Chandrika Casali: hair, Regis of Bruno Dessange; clothing, Thierry Mugler. Birgit Conrad: styling, Sylko. Mary Rita Schaub: hair, Max of Bumble & Bumble.

photo credits

Notes

Notes

Notes

Notes

Notes

Notes

Notes